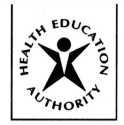

Health promotion in childhood and young adolescence for the prevention of unintentional injuries

**Elizabeth Towner, Gail Simpson
and Stephen Jarvis
Community Child Health
Department of Child Health
University of Newcastle upon Tyne
and
Therese Dowswell
Department of Psychology
University of Leeds**

**HEA Project Team
Jane Meyrick
and Antony Morgan**

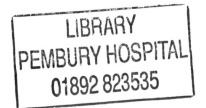

HEA Project Team
Jane Meyrick   Research Project Manager
Antony Morgan   Head of Monitoring and Effectiveness Research

Special thanks are due to Carol Sherriff and Lynne Friedli for
their commentaries.

This review was commissioned by the Health Education Authority
and carried out in collaboration with the NHS Centre for Reviews
and Dissemination, University of York.

In the same series:
Health promotion in older people for the prevention of CHD and
stroke
The effectiveness of video for health education

Forthcoming topics:
Young people and substance use
Young people and alcohol
Oral health
Healthy eating

For further information, tel. 0171 413 2624
To place an order, contact Marston Book Services, tel. 01235 465 565

9701200

WA 250

© Health Education Authority, 1996

ISBN 0 7521 0706 2

Health Education Authority
Hamilton House
Mabledon Place
London WC1H 9TX

Designed by Edwin Belchamber
Typeset by Wayzgoose
Cover design by Raymond Loewy International Ltd
Printed in Great Britain

Contents

Acknowledgements

During the preparation of the 1993 literature review we visited or telephoned a large number of people to seek their advice: their names are listed in Appendix F. We would very much like to thank them for their help. For the present review we would also like to thank the following people who sent us publications for inclusion: Dr B. Ytterstad, Ms Deirdre O'Reilly, Gordon Harland, Professor Jo Sibert. Dr Terry Klassen provided us with a copy of his MSc thesis, which was completed in May 1995 at McMaster University, Hamilton, Ontario: we would like to thank him for this useful contribution. We are also very grateful to Ms Alison Smith and Ms Pauline Leader for typing the report and tables, to Ms Ruth Bacon for collecting together the publications we have reviewed and to Phil Edwards and Ms Alison Avery for proofreading the manuscript.

This review includes some of the text of the 1993 HEA review; in other areas substantial revisions are made. We would like to thank the Health Education Authority for permission to include this information.

This review was carried out in collaboration with the NHS Centre for Reviews and Dissemination, University of York.

Structure of the report

The report begins with a commentary by Lynne Friedli, an Account Manager of the HEA, and Carol Sherriff, the Director of the Child Accident Prevention Trust, about why the review was commissioned and a discussion of some of the issues raised by the authors' conclusions about the research evidence presented.

The report is then divided into three main sections: executive summary, main report and technical appendices.

The *executive summary* contains the main findings; summary of findings from each area reviewed; recommendations for action and recommendations for future research.

The *main report* begins by providing background details about the review and the area of injury prevention including the methodology, definitions used and scope of the review. The report then presents all of the studies reviewed in detail, in Chapters 2 to 6.

The *technical appendices* present the authors' discussion of injury prevention and national policy initiatives, the scale of the problem, costs, mortality, morbidity and further discussion of the results of the review. They also include fuller details on methodology used in both this review and the review of reviews; a list of people consulted about the review; details of the search strategy and search times; the data extraction form; and a complete list of all the studies included. The report concludes with all the literature references.

Commentary

Carol Sherriff, Director, Child Accident Prevention Trust

Preventing unintentional injuries in childhood and young adolescence is an emotive subject which requires a rational and scientific response. It is difficult not to respond emotionally when 500–600 children die each year, 2.5 million attend an accident and emergency department and an uncounted number seek treatment from their GP as a result of an accident. These figures represent enormous physical, emotional and economic costs to children and young people, their families, friends, the NHS and society in general. However, 'accidents' are not random, haphazard events but are both predictable and preventable. Policymakers, purchasers and practitioners need to act upon that knowledge and base their decisions on injury data and on interventions which are shown to work.

This literature review is of significant assistance in that task. The review provides in one source information about the most effective forms of health promotion interventions. It provides policymakers, purchasers and practitioners with a clear guide to what has been demonstrated to reduce injury and change behaviour. It should be widely disseminated and urgently put into practice. That will not be easy. The interventions which are shown to work all rely on professionals and practitioners working across their disciplines, with parents and children and on a long-term basis. Such alliance working requires a sustained strategic approach and focused leadership. It invariably requires dedicated support for inter-agency collaboration and it must encourage the participation of parents and young people. All this, of course, requires the commitment of resources at national, regional and local level.

We should be aware of where the review cannot assist us. It contains little information about the cost of interventions, the process through which effective interventions are implemented and evaluated and the degree to which they have reduced the severity of injuries. This information is of crucial importance if we are to be able to replicate successful interventions. The review reminds us that we all have a role to play in documenting and evaluating our health promotion work.

It is disturbing that so little work has been done in certain areas of accident prevention. For example, there is little evidence of effective prevention in the play and leisure field although about 1.2 million children are injured in this area each year. Equally, older children/

younger adolescents, particularly those aged 9–14 years, are neglected in many intervention strategies. Yet this is a crucial time for young people moving from the close supervision of adults to a much greater degree of freedom. If we are to have a chance of influencing the behaviour of older adolescents, we cannot afford to miss this key group. Then, there is also the question of deprivation and unintentional injuries. The increasing study of this area is welcome, but the attention devoted to the link with deprivation does not begin to match the steep social gradient in mortality.

Finally, it is noticeable that some of the interventions listed show good evidence of behaviour change but none provides more than reasonable evidence of injury reduction. This is, of course, connected to the way in which studies are conducted and the use and availability of injury data. At a time when the health service is moving increasingly towards evidence-based medicine, we do need good evidence that interventions result in injury prevention and reduction. We also need information about the relative health impact of accidents and their prevention compared to the control and prevention of disease so that appropriate decisions can be made at local level. Policymakers, purchasers and practitioners can take the first steps in that direction by acting upon the recommendations in this review. I look forward to reading about their efforts in future reviews of effectiveness.

Commentary

Dr Lynne Friedli, Health Education Authority

As a leading provider of health promotion, the Health Education Authority is deeply committed to developing and disseminating expertise on effectiveness in the area of injury avoidance in young people. When the first edition of this study was published by the HEA in 1993, the evaluation of child accident prevention was a relatively undeveloped field, with little information to guide purchasers and practitioners. This valuable updated review considers the wealth of new studies available since then and demonstrates where there is sufficient evidence to merit immediate action in injury prevention.

The aim of the review is to focus energy and resources on those areas where there is reasonable or good evidence of effectiveness. While there is an ongoing need for further research in this area, notably in relation to cost effectiveness, there is an even more pressing need to ensure that current knowledge is widely disseminated. It is vital that planners, policy makers, professionals and the general public are aware of the valuable progress that has been made in assessing effectiveness and that the results of research are translated more rapidly into practice. This review makes a crucial contribution to this task.

The successful prevention of injuries to children and young people depends on a wide range of agencies and individuals working in partnership across professional boundaries. Healthy alliances provide a framework for developing a variety of approaches and the authors of this review stress the synergistic effect of combining different methods. Bringing together educational, environmental and legislative approaches does not mean the adoption of ad hoc measures, but the development of a complementary strategic approach. Such an approach requires leadership, dedicated support, training and time to bear results.

The Health Education Authority welcomes this review as a valuable resource to assist such a strategic approach to injury prevention. While the strongest evidence of effectiveness is in behaviour change, this is a crucial step in shifting the climate of public opinion and demonstrating that accidents are far from accidental.

Executive summary

Main findings

Multifactorial prevention
- Education, environmental modification and legislation all have a part to play and their effect in combination is important.

Injury prevention
- Examples of interventions which have been effective in reducing injury include: bicycle helmet legislation, area-wide traffic calming measures, child safety restraint legislation, child-resistant closures to prevent poisoning, window guards to prevent falls and domestic product design.

Behaviour change
- Interventions which have been effective in changing behaviour include bicycle helmet education and legislation, child restraint legislation, child restraint loan schemes, child restraint educational campaigns, pedestrian education aimed at the child and/or parent, provision of smoke detectors, and parent education on home hazard reduction.

- The capacity to bring about environmental and legislative change is often based on a climate of opinion resulting from educational campaigns.

Community-based interventions
- For the community-based campaigns we examined, the key to success was the sustained use of surveillance systems, the commitment to inter-agency co-operation and the time to develop networks and implement a range of interventions.

Implications for practice: what interventions work?
We have attempted to pull together evidence on effectiveness of different measures in the prevention of unintentional injury in childhood and adolescence. Within the tables we report which specific outcome measures were used in each study. Here we summarise the available state

of the evidence in two categories: behaviour change and injury reduction.

    ★   Some evidence
  ★★   Reasonable evidence
★★★ Good evidence

Interventions in the road environment
1. *General*
    Broad land use and transport policies   – little evidence
    Area-wide urban safety measure   – *injury reduction*★★

2. *Pedestrian injuries*
    Education/enforcement aimed at driver   – behaviour change★
    Education aimed at child/parent   – behaviour change★★
     – *injury reduction*★

3. *Bicycle injuries*
    Bicycle training   – little evidence
    Bicycle helmet educational campaigns   – behaviour change★★
    Bicycle helmet legislation   – behaviour change★★★
     – *injury reduction*★★

4. *Car passengers*
    Child restraint educational campaigns   – behaviour change★★
    Seat belt educational campaigns   – behaviour change★★
    Child restraint loan schemes   – behaviour change★★★
    Child restraint legislation   – behaviour change★★★
     – *injury reduction*★★

Interventions in the home environment
5. *General*
    Building regulations and home design   – little evidence
    Product design   – *injury reduction*★
    Safety devices   – *injury reduction*★

6. *Burns and scalds*
    Smoke detectors   – behavioural change★★
     – *injury reduction*★
    Tap water temperature reduction   – behavioural change★
     – *injury reduction*★
    Parent and child education   – behavioural change★

7. *Poisoning*
    Child-resistant packaging   – *injury reduction*★★
    Poisoning labelling   – little evidence
    Parent education   – behavioural change★

8. *Falls prevention*
    Window bars (education and   – behavioural change★★
    environmental modification
    and legislation)   – *injury reduction*★
    Parent education   – *injury reduction*★

9. *General campaigns*
    Parent education on hazard reduction   – behaviour change★★

Interventions in the leisure environment

10. *Drowning*
    Parent and child education   – behaviour change★
    Adult supervision of public swimming
    pools, beaches, etc.   – *injury reduction*★
                                 (little evidence)
    Pool design and protection   – *injury reduction*★

11. *Play and leisure injuries*
    Broad land use and transport policies   – little evidence, few
                                   studies
    Environment improvement – playground
    layout, equipment and surfacing   – little evidence
    Training schemes for adult supervision   – little evidence
    Protective equipment   – *injury reduction*★
                                   (little evidence)

Community-based studies
    Programmes targeting a range of injury   – behaviour change★★
    types in a range of different groups   – *injury reduction*★★

Summary of findings

1. The road environment

Broad land use and transport policies

- Policymakers need to recognise the impact that broad land use and transport policies have on childhood unintentional injury and act accordingly.

- Provision of school crossing patrols result in potential accident reduction.

Environmental modification of roads

- In Britain, area wide schemes resulted in a 13% reduction in accidental injuries

- Vulnerable road users such as child pedestrians and cyclists benefited from schemes.

Road safety education aimed at the driver
- Drivers are not prepared for the normal behaviour of child pedestrians and need to be more responsible in law for their actions.

- There are very few evaluated studies targeted at drivers.

- There is a strong relationship between the severity of pedestrian injuries and vehicle speed.

Road safety education aimed at the child
- There is a need for operational road safety programmes to have a sound empirical base – increasingly this has occurred in the studies published.

- Programmes need to be demonstrated to be effective in real road situations.

- Children's traffic clubs have shown mixed results, but injury reductions demonstrated elsewhere have not been replicated to such an extent in the UK.

- Parents need to be involved in pedestrian training programmes together with their young children.

- Lack of co-ordination between agencies has led to fragmented road safety education in the past.

Cycle helmets
- There is fairly strong evidence within the literature that it is possible to increase helmet wearing rates by concerted campaigns.

- There is growing evidence that increased wearing of cycle helmets leads to a reduction in injury rates.

Use of restraints – car occupants
- Legislation for restraint of children in cars has resulted in casualty reductions and should be extended.

- Seat belts and child restraints are effective if widely used and used correctly.

- Campaigns aimed at increasing seat belt use in older children have had mixed results; teenagers seem least amenable to change.

- Infant and child car restraints should be available to all and their widespread use promoted.

- Educational campaigns can be targeted at modifying policy and behaviour in institutions (e.g. child care centres) and these can be effective in changing parental behaviour.

2. The home environment

General home injuries

- Product improvements have led to injury reductions.

- A range of safety devices has been associated with lower risks: widespread use should be promoted.

- Home accidents encompass a wide range of injuries, causes and possible prevention strategies. Campaigns aimed at parents and children have mixed results.

- Window bars have resulted in a decrease in mortality due to falls.

- More data are needed on the links between home hazards and injury risk.

Fires, burns and scalds

- Safe home and product design remain important strategies to reduce risk of burn and scald injuries. Surveillance systems are important to enable rapid identification of those products associated with risk.

- The installation of smoke detectors in high-risk homes remains a target and a challenge for educators.

- There is a need for educational campaigns to increase awareness of the risks posed by hot water and kitchen hazards.

- There is a need for devices which regulate hot water temperature to be effective in everyday use.

Poisoning and suspected poisoning

- Child-resistant packaging of medicinal and non-medicinal agents has been shown to be effective to reduce poisoning injuries.

- 'Child-resistant' is not 'child-proof'. Safer packaging does not preclude the need for safe storage of hazardous substances.

- Campaigns aimed at raising awareness of home hazards have had mixed results.

- Parent education on the management of poisoning incidents is only partially effective.

3. The leisure environment

Drowning and near drowning
- For young children the risk of drowning in the bath is high. Educational campaigns need to continue to raise awareness of this risk.

- Garden ponds and domestic swimming pools pose a relatively large threat to young children considering the low level of exposure in England and Wales (Barry *et al.*, 1982; Kemp and Sibert, 1992). Adequate fencing regulations, complemented by public education have reduced this risk in other countries.

- Teaching children to swim is of protective value for older children.

- Adult supervision of public swimming pools enhances safety: the good safety record of indoor public pools must be safeguarded, and supervision of popular outdoor swimming amenities extended.

Play and sport injuries
- There was little evidence of evaluated interventions to reduce child injuries in the sport and leisure environment.

- Injury surveillance must underpin product and equipment re-design.

Community-based campaign
- Surveillance systems are important to provide local data to stimulate local interest, target specific injuries and age groups and to evaluate the impact of the programme.

- Inter-agency collaboration is essential to develop different elements of a local campaign

- Complementary use of educational, environmental and legislative approaches achieve the greatest success.

- Methods of cascade training using community volunteers are effective at a local level.

- Time is needed to develop the networks and range of local programmes.

- There is a need for the development of better outcome measures for evaluating the impact of local campaigns.

Recommendations for action

Combinations of methods. The synergistic effect of educational, environmental and legislative approaches needs to be stressed.

Healthy alliances have the potential to allow a variety of approaches to be developed and for these to complement and reinforce each other.

Educational approaches. Educational interventions need to be suited to the target group: the target group needs to be involved in the planning process. Participative rather than didactic approaches appear to have more success. One or two specific messages are preferable to a large number of messages and the inclusion of other specific groups such as parents or peers is useful. 'Expert' endorsement of a message by a doctor or health visitor for example has shown positive results.

Environmental modification. Encouragement of the wider use of small-scale environmental measures such as bicycle helmets or infant car seats needs to be reinforced by the low cost and easy availability of the safety device. A device also needs to be technologically sound.

Legislative approaches. In order to implement legislation, educational campaigns are needed to influence public opinion and policymakers.

Implications for purchasers
Purchasers within a district health authority need to consider the following:
- A long-term strategy and effective focused leadership for injury prevention.
- Dedicated support for inter-agency collaboration on injury prevention.
- More professional training in injury prevention.
- An advocacy role, e.g. for area-wide urban safety measures, improved product design, legislation.
- A direct role in increasing the availability of child car restraints through loan schemes, smoke detectors and bicycle helmets through educational campaigns and the encouragement of parent education of home hazard reduction.

Implications for policymakers
The issue of deprivation. What is notable about unintentional injury in childhood and early adolescence is the steep social gradient in mortality. Increasingly more attention has been paid in studies to the issue of deprivation. Examples of studies in which deprived groups or neighbourhoods have been targeted include the Safe Block project in Philadelphia (Schwarz *et al.*, 1993), the Safe Kids programme in Harlem (Davidson *et al.*, 1994), the Newcastle home safety study (Colver *et al.*,

1982), child restraint loan schemes targeted at low income families (Berger *et al.*, 1984), nurse practitioner poisoning counselling (Dershewitz and Paichel, 1984), and a nurse home visitation programme (Olds *et al.*, 1994).

The issue of deprivation and unintentional injury prevention needs to be a higher priority for policymakers.

Wider implementation of what is known. There are a number of areas where 'evidence of efficacy is sufficiently compelling to warrant immediate attempts to implement the specific preventive measures on the widest possible scale' (Pless, 1993). Policymakers need to be more aware of these areas and greater attention is needed on professional training for policymakers in the field of injury prevention.

Support for more emphasis on evaluation. The findings of this review reinforce the views of Foxcroft *et al.* (1996) who recommend that:

> a comprehensive policy change be implemented in the UK health promotion section which will result in more emphasis on evaluation, in recognition of the need to develop evidence based practice in health care and health promotion.

One recommendation is that more infrastructure support for evaluation should be provided locally through NHS R & D support units.

Recommendations for further research

Neglected areas of research
Some areas of injury prevention have very few evaluated studies. These include studies targeting the young adolescent age group and those targeting professionals or policymakers. There are very few evaluated studies in the areas of prevention of sports and leisure injuries. There is also potential in the application of behavioural methods including the use of rewards, the 'children helping children' approach (Morgan and Shute, 1990) and 'community mothers' approach (Johnson *et al.*, 1993), used in other areas of health education. The broad context of social, transport and land use policies is rarely addressed in relation to child and adolescent injury. The potential for further research in this field would appear to be high.

Improving the quality of research
More emphasis is needed on well designed and evaluated programmes, using randomised controlled designs where possible. For community-based programmes there have been difficulties designing studies because of the problem of experimentally controlling so many variables. More

attention is needed in this area, with greater attention paid to identifying suitable control groups. It is essential to develop good quality measures of non-fatal injury which include severity coding to use as outcome measures. There also needs to be research on the use of intermediate outcome measures such as risk data in evaluating programmes. Process details should be reported so that others can replicate interventions which have shown positive results, in other settings.

Regular updating of effectiveness reviews

This review has updated one carried out thirty months earlier and in the intervening period many new studies have been published. In addition during this time a new International Society for Child and Adolescent Injury Prevention has been formed, together with its journal *Injury Prevention*. The field of child and adolescent injury prevention is growing and maturing and this is reflected in the rate of increase in publications. There is a continued need for literature reviews on effectiveness in injury prevention to be updated regularly and for their findings to be disseminated to policymakers, researchers and practitioners.

1. Introduction

Background

In 1993 the Health Education Authority published *The effectiveness of health promotion interventions: a literature review* which concluded

> The whole area of injury prevention is still at an early stage of development – there is an urgent need for well-designed and evaluated studies to underpin the priority attached to this area in *The health of the nation* ...   (Towner *et al.*, 1993)

The aim of this publication is to critically review the world literature to provide information about the most effective forms of health promotion interventions in reducing childhood and adolescent (0–14 years) unintentional injury. The target audience is purchasers, practitioners (injury prevention co-ordinators, public health doctors, paediatricians, school nurses, health visitors, GPs), injury prevention academics and those responsible for policy at local and national levels. The review will also be of relevance to people in local authorities, voluntary organisations and community groups with interests in injury prevention.

Unintentional injury in childhood and young adolescence is a major public health problem in all developed and an increasing number of developing countries, but until the last decade it has received little attention at a national or international level. The prevention of accidents was identified as a key area in the *The health of the nation: a strategy for health in England* in 1992. The target for the 0–14 age group was to reduce the death rate by one third by the year 2005. To achieve such targets we need good information about effectiveness – in order to apply effective countermeasures more widely and to identify where gaps in knowledge occur.

Methodology

We identified relevant studies by a variety of methods: systematic searches of computerised databases, scanning the reference lists of other literature reviews and of important books and articles in the field, consultation with key informants and hand searching of journals. We obtained copies of relevant papers and a data extraction sheet was completed and each study was independently reviewed by two researchers. We included studies in which an injury prevention intervention had been evaluated and some outcome measures described.

We systematically extracted the data from the forms and summarised them in tables. The heterogeneity of injury types, study designs and statistical methodologies made a numerical synthesis of results impossible. Instead we have provided a narrative review.

A fuller description of the methodology used in this review is given in Appendix E, section 2.

Definitions

The review question

This review addresses the broad question: 'How effective are health promotion interventions in preventing unintentional injuries in childhood and young adolescence?'

The definition of *health promotion* we adopt is 'any planned measure which promotes health or prevents disease, disability and premature death' (Whitehead, 1991). It therefore encompasses health education, environmental modifications and legislation. In particular we examine preventive interventions in three environments: road, home and leisure, and in broader community-based programmes.

We have used Centre for Reviews and Dissemination guidelines in undertaking this review of the literature (Deeks *et al.*, 1995).

Age group

The age group of interest includes children and young adolescents aged 0–14 years, and their carers. This is not a homogeneous group: the type of accidents children have and where they occur reflect the child's age and stage of development and also their exposure to risk (of different hazards in different environments) at different ages (Towner and Jarvis, 1996).

Scope of the review

This publication updates and extends the previous review, includes papers that were not accessed in the first review and papers that have been published in the intervening 30 months. This review has been commissioned by the NHS Centre for Reviews and Dissemination, University of York and the Health Education Authority.

Since 1993 there have been considerable developments in the science and art of conducting effectiveness reviews, through developments in the

Cochrane Collaboration and the NHS Centre for Reviews and Dissemination (CRD). We seek to apply more rigour in the selection of studies for this publication and use CRD guidelines for carrying out systematic review of research (Deeks *et al.*, 1995). In addition we also attempt to conduct a 'review of reviews', pulling together the evidence from other reviews in this field that have been published in the last three years.

It addresses the broad question 'how effective are health promotion interventions in preventing unintentional injuries in childhood and young adolescence?' It examines the role of education, environmental modification and legislation and combinations of these approaches in injury prevention. Broader community-based studies are considered in detail.

2. The review of reviews

Further reviews of effectiveness have been published since the HEA literature review in 1993. Here we consider in more detail the nine reviews summarised in Table 2 using the methodology outlined in Appendix E, section 1. The recommendations of three of these are discussed more fully below.

Recommendations of other reviews on the effectiveness of interventions

Pless, I B. *The scientific basis of childhood injury prevention: a review of the medical literature* (Child Accident Prevention Trust, London, 1993)

Pless summarised the areas where evidence of efficacy is sufficiently compelling to warrant immediate action and this table is reproduced below from his review.

Injury type	Manoeuvre	Basis
Road – passenger	car seat restraint (expand and enforce legislation)	two group comparison studies: time series: quasi-experimental
Road – bicyclist	bike helmet (educate and legislate)	case control study of efficacy: two group before-and-after study of community intervention
Road – pedestrian	crossing guards; school zone speed restrictions; urban redesign	pre- and post-studies of urban redesigns; weak evidence for other recommended actions
Road – general	raise licensing and drinking age; lower speed limits; random breath testing (legislate)	two group comparison studies: time series: quasi-experimental
Burns	smoke detector (educate and legislate)	pre- and post-community intervention
Scalds	tap water temperature regulators (educate and legislate)	pre- and post-community intervention; two group comparisons
Drowning	pool fencing (regulate), learn-to-swim: life saving	pre- and post-surveys: no formal studies of other recommended actions

Home	window, fire, stair-guards	pre- and post-study of window guards: weak evidence for other recommended actions
Poisoning	child-resistant containers (enforcement)	pre- and post- and two group comparison studies
Leisure	playground standards (regulate and enforce)	pre- and post-surveys
Athletics	safety equipment regulations	no formal evaluations of recommended actions

Pless believed that part of the reason why very little information on effectiveness is used to its best advantage results from the fact that many potential participants have only taken 'bit roles' and there has been little co-ordinated activity.

Bass, J L, Christoffel, K K, Widome, M, Boyle, W, Scheidt, P, Stanwick, R and Roberts, K. Childhood injury prevention counseling in primary care settings: a critical review of the literature. *jx* **1993; 92(4): 544–80**

A panel of seven reviewers identified twenty articles which met their inclusion criteria. Of these 18 showed some positive effects of injury prevention counselling, including 15 which involved physician counselling. A variety of beneficial outcomes was reported: decreased hot water temperatures of tap water, increased use of car safety devices, increased use of seat belts.

Based on their review they recommend that counselling in primary care settings is an essential component of a comprehensive national strategy to prevent childhood injuries.

Klassen, T P. *The effectiveness of injury control interventions.* **(MSc thesis, McMaster University, Hamilton, Ontario, Canada, 1995)**

This included four systematic reviews : 1. randomised controlled trials of interventions in the home environment, 2. randomised controlled trials of interventions in the road environment, 3. school-based interventions, and 4. ambulatory care interventions. For home injury interventions, educational approaches proved to be effective at producing desired behavioural change but in the trials reviewed, the changes were accomplished by a one-time behavioural change and did not require a continuing process. In the road environment educational interventions were effective in producing behavioural change aimed at reducing injuries, although the effect waned over time.

Klassen found that there was evidence to support the use of safety programmes in schools: educational interventions within the school setting targeted at young children were effective in improving safety behaviour and in some case injury rates. The review also supported the view that clinicians should be involved in injury prevention. In the ambulatory setting, interventions were found to have a positive impact on safety behaviour; this held true for safety seat usage and home injury prevention but was not evident in bicycle helmet studies. For home injuries there was a trend which indicated that the more complex the action required, the less effective the intervention. Within the ambulatory care context it was important to prioritise those simpler actions which would achieve results. The review also highlighted the fact that for the adolescent age group there was very little evidence of effective intervention.

3. The road environment

The scale of the problem

Motor vehicle traffic accidents are a major cause of death and injury in childhood, accounting for just under half of all unintentional injury deaths. In 1992 in England and Wales 232 children were killed in road accidents: 64% of these as pedestrians, 19% as car occupants and 13% as cyclists. Boys were nearly twice as likely to be killed as girls. The difference is much more striking for cyclists: in 1992 all the deaths reported in the Department of Transport statistics were for boys. For car occupants the number of deaths for boys and girls are similar.

Road traffic accident statistics are compiled from police report forms (Stats 19). In 1992 36,674 children were reported as killed, seriously injured or slightly injured in road accidents (see Table 3); 232 of these were killed (1%), 6017 seriously injured (16%), and 30,425 (83%) slightly injured (see Home Office, 1993).

Child pedestrian accidents in Britain have been falling relative to the baseline of 1981–85, despite an increase of nearly 40% in the volume of traffic. In 1993 child pedestrian fatalities were 53% lower, those seriously injured 40% lower and slightly injured 24% lower. Some of this reduction may be related to lower pedestrian exposure with an increasing tendency for children to be transported by car (O'Reilly, 1994).

When British child casualty rates are compared with other countries in the Organisation for Economic Co-operation and Development (OECD), child pedestrian fatal casualty rates are amongst the worst and have been slower to decline than in comparable European Counties (O'Reilly, 1994). A Transport Research Laboratory paper looks at the factors relating to Britain's poor performance in child pedestrian casualties: levels of automation, exposure to traffic and remedial measures adopted in different countries may account for the differences (Lynam and Harland, 1992).

There is a steep social class gradient for road traffic accidents. There are four times as many pedestrian deaths in children in social class V than in social class I (OPCS, 1988). Child pedestrian casualty rates are highest in deprived inner city areas (Preston, 1972; King *et al.*, 1987). There is also some evidence that children from some ethnic groups may be more at risk. Lawson and Edwards (1991) found that young pedestrians (0–9 years) of Asian origin were overrepresented in childhood accidents in Birmingham by a factor of 2 but this could partly be explained by where the children live (inner city areas) and where road accidents occur.

When do accidents occur?

On weekdays 59% of fatal and serious child injuries take place between 8.00 am and 9.00 am and between 3.00 pm and 7.00 pm. These include journeys to and from school but also after school hours when children are involved in leisure activities (Jones, 1990). The winter months have the lowest number of child casualties, whilst the period from May to August has the highest.

Where do accidents occur?

Ninety-five per cent of child pedestrian and cyclist casualties occur in built-up areas and they tend to be scattered across the road network, rather than occur in clusters. Most are injured on minor rather than major roads. For children in cars, 75% of deaths occur in rural areas: the fatality rate on rural roads is $2\frac{1}{2}$ times higher than on urban roads, reflecting high traffic speeds (PACTS, 1992).

Exposure to injury risk

A study of pedestrian activity and accident risk in Northampton, England, confirms that 'the risk to children on all parts of the road network is higher than that for adults' and also brings new insights into the vulnerability of pedestrians of different ages (Ward *et al.*, 1994). Boys aged 5–15 years are one-and-a-half times more at risk of being injured than girls in this age group. However when exposure is taken into account boys and girls aged 5–9 have very similar casualty rates per kilometre walked. For older girls (aged 10–15) a different picture emerges: they appear to be less able than boys of this age to walk alongside or cross the road safely.

> Indeed girls of this age have the highest casualty rates of any age group for both kilometres walked alongside traffic and for roads crossed.
>
> (Ward *et al.*, 1994)

The findings of this report have important policy implications about the safety of the pedestrian environment.

Prevention

Broad land use and transport policies

Although individual behaviour does have a part to play, land use and transport policies have a significant impact on children's use of the road environment, both for play and for moving from place to place. These policies also affect the nature (e.g. public/private), volume and speed of traffic. Whitelegg (1987) describes a road traffic accident as being:

> a function of the land use system, residential patterns, population densities, street geometry, location of workplace, shopping precinct, health centre or other traffic generators.

What is more difficult to demonstrate is how these policies directly affect child casualties on the roads. A journey made by car, for example, is three times more likely to injure a pedestrian than a journey made by bus (Transport & Health Study Group, 1991). The removal of subsidies for public transport in London by the Greater London Council was associated with increased road casualties (Allsop et al., 1987). A greater emphasis on public rather than private transport could potentially reduce road traffic accidents.

Differences in child casualty rates occur in different housing areas. King et al. (1987) found lower child accident casualties in post-war housing estates than in streets of Victorian terraced houses with little or no garden, few garages and much on-street parking. They recommend that road safety should be one of the objectives of environmental improvement and that the density of child accidents in inner city areas should be one of the criteria used in the selection of improvement areas.

Transport policies also have many other wide-ranging impacts on risk exposure and injury rates. For instance perceived risk of accidents can restrict children's independent mobility. Hillman et al. (1990) found that over the period 1971 to 1990 the 'licences' adults gave their children had decreased. Parents were reacting to the dangers in the road environment and escort journeys had risen dramatically during this time from 14% to 64%. These additional escort journeys could further exacerbate the risk to other vulnerable road users by increasing the volume of traffic.

Transport policies also determine the provision of school crossing patrols. A study of the effectiveness of school crossing patrols in Buckinghamshire demonstrated that the provision of patrols at sites meeting local authority criteria resulted in accident reductions (Boxall, 1988); see Table 4.

International comparisons can provide some indication of potential health gain from major environmental and policy change. For children under the age of 10 years, the death rate for road traffic accidents is three times as high in the United Kingdom as in Sweden and for the 10–14 age group the United Kingdom pedestrian death rate is one of the worst in Europe (Preston, 1992; Department of Transport, 1990). Pedestrian and cycling exposure to the road environment appears to vary considerably in different European countries. Per head of population

Britain has a low cycling fatality rate, but in terms of cycling fatalities per kilometre cycled, Britain has a worse cycling accident record than Denmark, the Netherlands and Germany (Mynors and Savell, 1992). More studies of pedestrian and cycling exposure are needed in different countries before meaningful comparisons can be made. Both the Netherlands and Germany have experienced very large reductions in child pedestrian casualty rates over the last 15 years, far greater than those achieved in the United Kingdom (Lynam and Harland, 1992). The implication remains that Britain has the potential to reduce its pedestrian and cycling casualties to the level of the safest in Europe.

Environmental modification of roads

Area-wide urban safety measures

Children's accidents on urban roads are widely scattered across the whole road network and do not occur in clusters or 'blackspots', where high-risk site measures can be applied. During the 1970s and 1980s a number of countries have introduced experimental area-wide urban safety measures aimed at reducing accidents to vulnerable road users such as pedestrians and cyclists. Pharoah and Russell (1989) describe a number of schemes in three European countries.

The urban safety schemes included a package of measures tailored to suit the needs of individual areas. A hierarchy of roads was designated for a town in which roads for through traffic were identified; the areas which were normally residential were modified to incorporate measures to reduce speed and volume of traffic (Ward, 1991).

Table 5 lists studies from Denmark, Germany, the Netherlands and Britain where urban safety demonstrations have been conducted. All these studies relate to large scale area-wide schemes, conducted over a long period of time. The Netherlands study, for example, was conducted over 15 years: a 6-year 'before' period of data collection, 4 years when measures were introduced and a 5-year 'after' period of data collection. An interesting feature of the Netherlands' scheme in Rijswijk and Eindhoven was the comparison of the effectiveness of three packages of road safety measures. Package 1 included very simple measures to exclude through traffic from residential areas. Package 2 included more extensive measures to exclude most local traffic and to limit the speed of remaining traffic. Package 3 was a complete reconstruction of areas as pedestrian priority areas on the Woonerf model (redesign of the road environment to give pedestrians priority as used in the Netherlands). The second of these packages reduced injuries by up to 25% (Janssen, 1991). Other European studies report a number of successful outcomes but often too few details are provided to evaluate the results adequately.

As conditions vary from country to country, we look in more detail at the Urban Safety Project which has been conducted in Britain by the Transport and Road Research Laboratory (Lynam *et al.*, 1988). Locality areas in Reading (Ward *et al.*, 1989a), Sheffield (Ward *et al.*, 1989b), Nelson (Walker and Gardner, 1989), Bradford (Walker and McFetridge, 1989) and Bristol (Ward *et al.*, 1989c) were selected, each with about 100 road traffic accidents involving injury per annum, together with paired control areas of similar characteristics. Measures to redistribute traffic and improve the safety of individual roads were introduced; for example more roundabouts, banned right turns, closures of roads, sheltered parking, right-turn bays and a series of central refuges on wider roads to reduce speeds, discourage overtaking and aid pedestrians.

Outcome was judged by changes in Stats 19 road traffic accident injury rates over a 7-year period (5 years before and 2 years after implementation of measures (Mackie *et al.*, 1988, 1990). Table 5 shows that overall accident reduction of 13% occurred (all ages and all types of injury) attributable to the schemes but that there were great variations between schemes. Slight accidents declined proportionately more than fatal and serious ones. Pedestrian injuries were reduced particularly in Sheffield and there was a general reduction in child cyclist casualties. The measures that were particularly successful were those that protected two-wheeled vehicles (such as right-turn prevention, right-turn bays and central road dividers).

Each scheme cost about £250,000 and first-year rates of return indicated considerable accident cost savings (Mackie *et al.*, 1990). The interim results from Reading showed accident reductions of between 4% and 15%: an assessment of a further five years' data suggests that child pedestrians and cyclists benefited more particularly from the scheme in the longer term (Tillman, 1992).

Lessons learnt in the United Kingdom and elsewhere are now incorporated in a strategy for urban safety management which encompasses a multi-disciplinary approach (Institute of Highways and Transportation, 1990). Ward points out that local area safety schemes only work effectively if the help and co-operation of local people have been established both in setting the agenda and in implementation and use (Ward, 1991).

Road safety education aimed at the driver

Education/enforcement aimed at the driver
Two opposing views (King *et al.*, 1987) of a road traffic accident are
- a pedestrian masked by a stationary vehicle, and
- a driver travelling too fast to see a pedestrian.

Thompson *et al.* (1985) measured vehicle speeds outside junior schools in Nottingham and recorded the cars' distances from the kerb. The presence of children by the roadside had no effect on the drivers' speed or position in the road. Even large groups of pedestrians only reduced mean speeds by one mile per hour. The authors concluded that vehicle drivers were inadequately prepared for the unpredictable behaviour of child pedestrians.

Howarth and Gunn (1982) argue the case for making drivers more responsible in law for their actions. Preston (1990) supports this view in her promotion of Home Zones where, in small residential areas, child pedestrians should have priority and any driver who injures a child should be presumed negligent.

A programme in Canada has targeted both drivers and pedestrians (Malenfant and Van Houten, 1989); see Table 6. The 'Courtesy Promotes Safety' Programme included education, engineering and enforcement in its pedestrian safety programme to increase the safety of pedestrians at cross walks on a city-wide basis. Feedback signs reported percentages of motorists yielding to pedestrians each week. The programme produced increases in percentage of motorists yielding right of way to pedestrians.

The speed at which a car is driven has a strong relationship to the severity of pedestrian injuries. When pedestrians are struck by a moving car, at 20 mph only 5% are killed, at 30 mph 45% are killed and this rises to 85% killed at 40 mph (Kimber, 1990). The Department of Transport has published a strategy for tackling the problems of excessive speed which includes both traffic calming and changing drivers' attitudes towards speeding (Department of Transport, 1992).

Road safety education aimed at the child

Road safety education – experimental programmes (Table 7)
Rivara *et al.* (1991) have estimated that road crossing can involve up to 26 different tasks to negotiate traffic successfully. Most of the pedestrian training schemes listed in Table 7 focus on a small number of these, for example, finding a safe place to cross, improving road timing skills and making effective use of gaps between traffic or very specific crossing situations such as mid-block dart-outs (children running out on to roads in straight stretches of roads, not at intersections, i.e. in the middle of a block). The studies are all small-scale, involve children below the age of 10 years, and measure knowledge and/or behaviour before and after the training programme.

Sandels (1975) in her work on child pedestrian behaviour in Sweden concluded that:

> it is not possible to adapt fully young children to the traffic environment. They are biologically incapable of managing its many demands.

Thomson *et al.* (1992) do not support this view and consider that practical training programmes, properly targeted on relevant and clearly defined road crossing skills, have considerable potential. In their programmes of training children to find safe places to cross, Thomson and his colleagues have found few differences in children's knowledge between roadside instruction and classroom training with the use of table top models. A number of the published studies report significant knowledge or observed behaviour improvements on simulated roads following training, which are maintained over a period of time (Yeaton, 1978). Observations were not made on young children crossing real roads.

In these experimental studies most involve very few agencies, the researchers chiefly working with the children through schools. Some of the studies however included parents as well as their children: Rivara *et al.* (1991) found that improved performance in observed pedestrian skills of children crossing real roads, occurred when a parental component was included. In the Netherlands van der Molen *et al.* (1983) actively involved parents of pre-school children in a pedestrian training programme for their children and found that parents subsequently set better examples to the children they accompanied and gave more verbal instructions. Adult road crossing strategies are markedly different from those that road users are taught and demand highly developed perceptual and motor skills (Thomson, 1991).

Operational programmes – traffic clubs

Traffic clubs have been organised in a number of countries. In the United Kingdom the Tufty Club was used by parents of pre-school children and in schools. Firth (1973) found improvements in road safety knowledge, but a later assessment of the effectiveness of the clubs in Lancashire found no evidence that the Tufty Club had contributed anything to children's knowledge of road safety (Antaki *et al.*, 1986); see Table 8.

In the late 1960s in Norway, children's traffic clubs were developed with the aim of reducing child casualties by improving road safety by practical instruction and training by parents. Children were enrolled by parents on their third birthday and traffic education was distributed to parents on a six-monthly basis. Schioldborg (1976) evaluated the clubs by assessing road safety knowledge, behaviour and accident rates. The results reported appear impressive with members having 20% lower accident rates than non-members and in Oslo the rates were 40% lower for members. However, only one-third of the eligible children joined the clubs and Grayson (1981) has pointed out the methodological problems of selective membership: was the difference due to the beneficial effects of the clubs or the characteristics of the families who joined the clubs? (Grayson, 1981). Similar traffic clubs have been introduced in other Scandinavian countries, Germany and Luxembourg. In the United Kingdom, the Streetwise Kids Club was introduced in London, but membership was low, and particularly so in lower social class groups (Downing, 1987).

A more recent evaluation of the Eastern Region Traffic Club (sponsored by a commercial insurance company) showed increased membership (49% of relevant age group) with all social groups represented. Initial findings showed some improvements in parents' knowledge and reported behaviour among club members.

An evaluation by West *et al.* (1993) showed that the Traffic Club reduced the incidence of children running on ahead of parents when out walking, but there was no effect on whether children crossed the road alone, played unsupervised in the street or rode bicycles unsupervised. The first evidence of the Traffic Club's impact on casualty reduction is now available (Bryan-Brown, 1995). Twenty per cent reductions have been observed in casualties involving children emerging from behind a vehicle in the intervention area of the Eastern Region (Bryan-Brown, 1995).

While in the UK the Traffic Club appears to have some positive effects on both behaviour and casualty reduction, the more recent evidence from Sweden is more negative. Gregersen and Nolen (1994) examined the accident risks of members and non-members of the Swedish Traffic Club and found that members reported significantly higher traffic accident risk. This would suggest that the Traffic Club was ineffective and possibly harmful but these results could possibly be due to differential reporting bias by club members.

Operational programmes – other programmes

In the UK, the Green Cross Code has been widely used since its introduction in the early 1970s. The code was based on a consensus of information from mothers, road safety officers and teachers and the wording was carefully piloted with young children (Sargent and Sheppard, 1974). The code's introduction was associated with a reduction of 11% in child pedestrian accidents. An Organisation for Economic Co-operation and Development report on mass media (OECD, 1978) singled out the Green Cross Code as the only proven measure in the road safety literature. It has been questioned, however, whether this reduction was a direct result of the code or the publicity campaign which accompanied it, or whether it was connected with the energy crisis when there was general reduction in road accidents (Grayson and Howarth, 1982; Thomson, 1991).

In the USA, Preusser and Blomberg (1984) developed the Willy Whistle public information and education materials designed to reduce one specific but common injury type, 'mid-block dart and dash accidents', in 3- to 8-year-old children. Films, posters and television slots were produced and distributed widely in three cities. Behavioural observations showed that children crossed more carefully and there were 21% reductions in mid-block dash accidents with a 31% reduction in the 5–6 age group. The authors felt that the Willy Whistle campaign resulted from a process which combined research, evaluation and media production and that the process was,

> driven by accident data that were used to define the problem and structure the solution.

The programme had little or no effect on reducing casualties in older children. Preusser and Lund (1988) later developed a pedestrian safety education film entitled *'And Keep Looking'* aimed at 9- to 12-year-old children with a more sophisticated message reflecting the older children's greater independent use of the road environment. The film's impact was evaluated in several cities and produced improvements in knowledge and behaviour and reductions in casualties. Casualty reductions have not been replicated in other areas outside the study.

In the UK the 'Let's Decide Walk Wise' programme is an operational programme which has developed from the experimental programmes devised by Ampofo-Boateng *et al.* (1992) and Thomson *et al.* (1992). The school-based pedestrian training resource for 5- to 8-year-old children has practical sessions in the road environment, work using a table top model and curriculum work in the classroom. Children were tested on their choice of safe routes using a table top model and the programme appeared to be partially effective. Outside parent helpers were used for the practical work in the road environment and those schools that complied with the designed programme proved more effective than the less compliant schools (Harland and Tucker, 1994).

This finding was also observed in the evaluation of the Streets Ahead programme in Australia: the schools which practised crossing behaviour at real sites showed greater improvements in children's crossing behaviour (Penna and Lambert, 1994). This evaluation included the observation of children's road crossing behaviour by video. Another interesting Australian programme, the Safe Routes to School programme attempts to tailor educational and engineering initiatives to the traffic problems identified in individual schools (Tziotis, 1994). The only evaluation reported is a small-scale one and the author recommends more extensive evaluation be conducted using methods similar to those developed by Penna and Lambert (1994).

The range of methods used in the 'Let's Decide Walk Wise', Streets Ahead and Safe Routes to School programmes, involving both practical and teaching sessions and tailoring environmental measures to the local school, contrast with the one-off lecture approach of the 'Think First' Programme reported from the United States (Wright *et al.*, 1995). This latter programme was aimed at reducing brain and spinal cord injuries in youth and attempted to cover a wide range of topics in a very short period. The programme proved to be ineffective and possibly harmful.

An evaluation of cycle training in Cambridgeshire for 8- to 10-year-olds showed both playground and road trained groups performing significantly better than a control group on right and left turns in a real road environment (Traffic and Road Research Laboratory, 1980).

In the Netherlands van Schagen and Brookhuis (1994) compared two training methods to teach young cyclists to behave correctly at intersections in their interactions with traffic. One method includes theory and practical training and the second just practical training. The authors concluded that neither method was very effective and their observations led them to believe that children applied informal rather than formal rules when dealing with traffic and these informal rules should be used as the starting point for training activities.

Grayson and Howarth (1982) have maintained that:

> the assessment of wide ranging educational principles is a far more difficult task than the evaluation of some traffic engineering measures.

Singh and Spear (1989) conducted a comprehensive review during the mid-1980s of road safety education in the United Kingdom in schools and colleges and also assessed the involvement of the police, road safety officers and the local education authorities. They identified the lack of a properly developed organisational structure, poor co-ordination of agencies and lack of initial teacher training. Stimulated by the review, the Transport Road Research Laboratory developed a code of good practice in road safety education in schools (Harland *et al.* 1991). Both this, and the local authority association's Road Safety Code of Good Practice call for a more co-ordinated approach by the agencies involved. A local authority-based demonstration project in Sheffield and Hertfordshire is currently testing good practice in road safety education and is being evaluated by Singh *et al.* (Harland, 1992).

Cycle helmets

Background

In the last two years three reviews have discussed evidence related to cycle helmets and strategies to promote cycle helmet wearing. Hillman (1993) looks at the case for and against cycle helmets and makes the important point that promoting cycle helmet wearing shifts the responsibility from the car driver to the cyclist; cyclists do not often drive into cars, it is usually cars which drive into cyclists. The Transport Research Laboratory review of cycle helmets has drawn upon 54 papers: it examines the effect of cycle helmets in reducing head injuries, the strategies used to increase helmet wearing, attitudes to helmets and cycle helmet wearing rates (Royles, 1994) . The third review by Graitcer et al. (1995) reviews educational and legislative strategies to promote bicycle helmets. These reviews are a useful source of additional information to that provided below.

Cycle injuries. Road traffic accident data collected by the police (Stats 19 data) for 1992 (Department of Transport, 1993) show that 31 children under the age of 15 years were killed as a result of pedal cycle injuries, 934 were seriously injured and 5276 were slightly injured in England and Wales (see Table 3). Department of Transport (1993) figures show that 4.3 pedal cyclists (all ages) were killed for every 100 million kilometres of road in 1992. At least two-thirds of cyclists killed in accidents had head injuries which contributed to or resulted in death of the cyclist (Royles, 1994).

Bicycle helmet wearing rates. Research International UK in 1993 (see Royles, 1994) reported a large increase in helmet ownership among junior and secondary-school children. Junior-school children's ownership of helmets rose from 13% in 1991 to 39% in 1993 and those who always wore a helmet increased from 2% to 11% over this time period. These figures are similar to those from a survey of 4637 secondary-school children in Newcastle in 1990: 4% of 11- to 12-year-olds reported wearing a cycle helmet the last time they rode a bicycle compared with 2% of 13- to 14-year-olds; 4% of boys compared with 2% of girls had worn a helmet (Towner et al., 1994).

Studies of cycle helmet strength. The physical strength of helmets is important when considering if helmets prevent different types of injuries. Helmets of approved standards are protective for the majority of accidents where the head is hit but they cannot protect the head in a high velocity direct impact (Mills, 1989).

Cyclist risk assessment

Dorsch et al. (1987) conducted a postal survey of members of cycling clubs in Australia. In all 1321 people were contacted, 894 responded and 197 gave details of accidents sustained in the previous 5 years where there had been some head impact. A statistically significant association between helmet use and reduced head injury severity was demonstrated and Dorsch *et al.* concluded 'the risk of death from head injury is 3–10 times greater for unhelmeted relative to helmeted bicyclists'. A widely cited case control study in Seattle calculated that riders with helmets had an 85% reduction in their risk of head injuries and an 88% reduction in the risk of brain injuries. This study design may be limited because helmet wearers may take fewer risks or have less exposure to cycling and thus less likelihood of serious accident (McCarthy, 1991). There are other limitations to this research resulting from differences in the cases, and/or the controlled population groups (Thompson *et al.*, 1989 discussion; Royles, 1994).

Spaite *et al.*(1991) evaluated the impact of helmet use on injury severity and found that non-users of helmets were in higher impact crashes than helmet users and injuries suffered in other body areas were more severe. They concluded that some of the 'protection' afforded helmet wearers could be explained by safer riding habits. Maimaris *et al.* (1994) compared injury patterns of cycle helmet wearers and non-wearers attending an accident and emergency department in the UK and found an increased risk among the non-wearers of sustaining head injury in a bicycle accident when a motor vehicle was involved. In both this UK study and one from Australia (Thomas *et al.*, 1994) the protective effect of helmet wearing for bicycle accidents was confirmed.

Debate about the benefits of helmets for cyclists continues (Trippe, 1992). Anti-helmet campaigners argue that cycle helmets do not improve safety but place responsibility for injury protection on the victim (McCarthy, 1992). Pro-helmet campaigners believe that helmets are an effective safety measure and their widespread use should be promoted (Illingworth, 1992). The test, however, of the true effectiveness of cycle helmets is whether community-wide promotion of cycle helmets has had any impact on casualty or severity reduction.

Evaluation of the impact of cycle helmet programmes

A number of studies have evaluated the effect of a programme on increasing bicycle helmet wearing rates (the impact of a programme). During the 1980s campaigns have taken place in Australia, Canada and the USA (see Table 9). Several studies have reported positive outcomes as far as increased helmet wearing is concerned. Most of these studies recorded before and after *observed* helmet wearing rates in target populations. A small number of studies described a favourable outcome in terms of *reported* helmet wearing rates or increased knowledge amongst the target populations. A few studies describe poor outcomes from campaigns, including a study of an intervention specifically aimed at children who had already sustained injuries as a result of a bicycling accident. The national Safe Kids campaign in the United States promoted helmet campaigns in its state and local level coalitions (Mickalide, 1991). Sales and ownership of helmets increased but no decrease in injuries was mentioned.

The Seattle bicycle helmet campaign included the main elements which characterised the most successful interventions (Bergman *et al.*, 1990). First, there was a fairly tight focus in terms of the target age group. Second the campaign had a single aim – increased rates of helmet wearing. Third, the campaign drew together a range of organisations and individuals (health professionals, teachers and businesses), used a variety of locations (for example, schools and physicians' offices) and a range of educational methods (from mass media to targeted one-to-one counselling). Last, it addressed the issue of cost by various subsidies.

The campaign resulted in an increase in observed helmet wearing rates amongst the target population from 5% to 14%, as compared with an increase from 1% to 4% in the control group. However a single comparison area was used and the control and study populations were not comparable for helmet use at the start of the study.

A schools bicycle helmet promotion programme in Canada was more successful in schools in high income areas compared with schools in low income areas (Parkin *et al.*, 1993). A community-wide campaign initiated by a coalition of volunteers in the United States found that two specific campaign components appeared to have the greatest influence on child helmet ownership receiving advice from a physician and receiving advice over the telephone (Schneider *et al.*, 1993). However, other sources of information, such as direct mail and a bicycle rodeo were not associated with child helmet ownership.

The process of developing an educational programme to promote bicycle helmet wearing is well documented by Stevenson and Lennie (1992) in Queensland, Australia but this programme was not evaluated. Emphasis was given to a participative form of action research using focus groups and workshops. Strikingly different rates of bicycle helmet wearing occurred between primary and high school students and barriers to helmet wearing were extensively explored. While the programme was being developed the Queensland government announced that helmet wearing would be made compulsory. In addition, a non-interventionist strategy was advocated by the students and so the programme was not evaluated.

The passage of a bicycle helmet law (the first of its kind in the United States) provided Dannenberg *et al.* (1993) with the opportunity to compare legislation and educational approaches. They found that legislation combined with education was more effective than education alone in modifying children's behaviour in relation to bicycle helmet use. Self-reported helmet use in the legislation county (Howard County) rose from 11% to 38% after the law and educational campaign compared with Montgomery County where educational efforts were undertaken (8% to 13% and from 7% to 11% in the comparison county of Baltimore County (no education or legislation) (Dannenberg *et al.*, 1993); see Table 10.

Evaluation of outcome of programmes

A smaller number of studies have gone on to examine whether increased helmet wearing has affected health outcomes. The strongest evidence for promoting cycle helmet wearing comes from Victoria , Australia, and there are many lessons in this campaign from which we can learn (see Table 10).

In July 1990 the state of Victoria, Australia introduced the first law in the world requiring cyclists to wear helmets. This was preceded by a decade of helmet promotion. A good series of observational studies of helmet wearing over a number of years have been carried out in Melbourne and more widely in Victoria and it has been possible to document bicycle head injuries through both hospital admissions and emergency attendance data and through insurance company claims. Because of the preceding 10 years of promotional campaigns to increase helmet wearing, we are able to consider a much wider time frame rather than just examining helmet wearing rates and head injury rates before and after the law was passed.

The health promotion campaigns which preceded the law included education, mass media publicity, support by professional associations and community groups, consultations with community groups and financial incentives. Cameron *et al.* (1992) point out that a climate of opinion favourable to the introduction of bicycle helmet legislation had been created in Victoria in the 1960s and the 1970s, through the introduction of motorcycle helmet law, compulsory seat belts, child restraint laws, random breath tests and engine capacity limits for novice motorcyclists. During the 1980's a decade of health promotion activities took place to increase helmet use. The health promotion activities are discussed in detail by Cameron *et al.* (1994) and Leicester *et al.* (1991) but some of the activities relating to children are described here. In 1980 a bicycle safety education unit (Bike Ed) for use by students aged 9–13 years was developed. Promotion of helmets was conducted by this unit in schools. A mass media campaign targeted primary-school students in 1984 and rebate schemes were introduced. There was wide consultation with cycling groups and work on helmet standards. Enforcement of the law was relatively modest: for children this involved a bicycle offence report being sent to their parents. Cameron *et al.* (1994) comment:

> if a community understands the benefits of a safety measure, and a reasonable proportion has already been persuaded to adopt it voluntarily, then considerably increased use can be achieved through a law, even with relatively moderate levels of enforcement.

Helmet wearing rates in Victoria rose from 5% in 1982/83 to 31% in 1989/90 to 75% in 1991 following introduction of the legislation. However legislation was also accompanied by a decrease in cycling in some groups. In Melbourne observations of cycling suggests that following legislation there was no reduction in adult cyclist exposure, moderate effects on children (aged 5–11 years where 10% less were observed cycling) and great effects on teenagers (12–17 years) in whom a 46% decrease was observed (Finch *et al.*, 1993).

There was a significant post-law increase in helmet wearing rates in all three groups. Children's (5–11 years) wearing rates increase from 65% pre-law, to 78% in 1991 and 77% in 1992. Teenagers' (12–17 years) wearing rates increased from 21% pre-law to 45% in 1991 and 59% in 1992 and adults from 36% pre-law to 74% in 1991 and 84% in 1992.

Observations in 1991 revealed that 20% of teenagers carried rather than wore helmets but a year later compliance was much higher and only 6% were observed carrying their helmets when riding (Finch *et al.*, 1993).

In Victoria there was a reduction of 48% in head injured admissions or deaths between 1989/90 and 1990/91 and a 70% decrease between 1989/90 and 1990/91. This was accompanied by a reduction in non-head injuries of 23% in the first period and 28% in the second. During this period there were also a number of other safety initiatives in Victoria including drink driving campaigns and speeding campaigns which would have resulted in fewer crashes.

In summary the introduction of legislation was accompanied by immediate large reductions in the number of cyclists with head injuries. This was achieved through reductions in the number of cyclists involved in crashes, partly through decrease in bicycle use and partly from the reduction in the risk of head injury of cyclists involved in crashes.

Use of restraints – car occupants

There is considerable evidence that child seat restraints (for young children) when properly used, reduce car occupant injuries (Christian and Bullimore, 1989; Agran *et al.*, 1987). The problem for health promoters has been how to get widespread use and correct use of child seat restraints. There are two main strategies: (a) legislation, and (b) campaigns of education and loan schemes. In this section we also consider (c) child education programmes to increase seat belt use in older children.

Child restraint legislation (see Table 11)

There have been various studies reporting the effects of child restraint legislation in the United States as summarised in Table 11. Much of this legislation applies only to children under 4. Many of the evaluations report positive results both in terms of observed restraint use by those children covered by the legislation and reductions in injuries and deaths. Decker *et al.* (1984) reported a 50% decrease in fatalities of children under 4 as a result of legislation in Tennessee.

Few authors report significant increases in observed restraint use by those children not covered by the law (children over 4) (e.g. Agran *et al.*, 1987). However legislation in the USA has not resulted in universal compliance, restraint usage rates of 40–50% are reported. An inter-state comparison by Seekins *et al.* (1988) suggested that the greater the enforcement effort, the higher the compliance, and Agran *et al.* (1987) concluded that despite legislation

> there remains a large number of children seen in the emergency room who are unrestrained despite the enactment of a child passenger safety law,

and called for education campaigns to increase correct restraint use. Dejeammes *et al.* (1986) studied the effectiveness of child restraint laws in 17 countries: they found that child restraint usage rates in the countries with laws are not usually at the levels reached for adult belts.

Lessons from the United States and other countries might not be totally relevant to the British context. Seat belt legislation in Britain for adult front seat passengers led to much higher compliance than similar legislation in the United States (Mackay, 1987, Williams and Lund, 1987). Lowne *et al.* (1984) reviewed the effect of United Kingdom seat belt legislation on restraint usage by children. They found that following the 1983 introduction of compulsory use of restraints for front seat occupants of passenger cars, there was little overall effect on the numbers of fatal and serious injuries in children; except in the 11 to 14 age group where there was a marked reduction in injuries to children travelling in the front seat. The Child Accident Prevention Trust (1988) also conducted a useful review of the safety of children in cars. In Britain, legislation was introduced in 1989 making it compulsory for children under 14 to be restrained when in the rear of a car *provided a restraint was available*. In 1989 the number of children using rear seat belts increased from 45% to 78% (Department of Transport, 1990). In April 1992 observed restraint use by rear seat belt occupants in two study areas in Crowthorne and Nottingham was 88% in children under one year, 84% in the 1–4 age group, 71% in the 5–9 age group and 60% in the 1013 age group (TRL, 1992). There is no published evidence of the effect of this legislation on casualty reduction.

Infant restraint promotion campaigns (Tables 13 and 14)
There have been evaluations of child restraint loan schemes in the USA, New Zealand, Australia, the United Kingdom and Sweden. The

campaigns to increase correct restraint use include educational sessions, restraint rental schemes and the provision of free infant seats. Results of evaluated studies are summarised in Table 13.

Several educational campaigns (Reisinger, 1978; Goodson, 1985; Geddis, 1982) and infant seat loan schemes (e.g. Colletti, 1986) have reported increases in observed correct usage of infant restraints, although in some cases inappropriate usage was also increased (Berger, 1984; Downing and Franklin, 1989). Initial improvements in restraint usage were not always sustained over time (Geddis, 1982) and gains were sometimes modest (Reisinger, 1981) especially in schemes in low income communities (Berger, 1984; Robitaille *et al.*, 1990); see Table 14.

An evaluation of infant restraint loan schemes in Britain reported modest improvements in the numbers of infants observed correctly restrained in cars (Downing and Franklin, 1989). Correctly restrained infants increased from 8% to 16% but there were also increases in infants transported in non-approved devices, such as carry cots which increased from 11% to 23%. At hospital discharge in the United Kingdom 'most babies still sit on their mothers' laps in the rear' and Downing and Franklin (1989) called for a review of hospital policy relating to this.

Restraint promotion amongst older children (see Table 14)
Downing and Franklin (1989) also monitored restraint use by older children and reported low restraint use on school journeys by children travelling in the rear of cars. Despite partial legislation, many children travel in cars inadequately restrained. Several campaigns encouraging children to 'buckle up' have been reported and have met with mixed success. An educational programme aimed at teenagers resulted in increased knowledge but no changes in attitudes or behaviour of these older children (Neuwelt, 1989); see Table 14.

A programme in the USA by one paediatrician aimed at increasing seat belt use in school age children resulted in observed seat belt use increasing by 38% but the improvement was not sustained over time (Macknin *et al.*, 1987). The Bucklebear programme used in day-care centres and nursery schools was successful in increasing children's use of safety seats or seat belts (Chang *et al.*, 1985) A community-wide programme reported by Roberts and Fanurik (1986) to increase seat belt use by primary-school aged children, increased use from 4–5% before the campaign to 66–70% during the campaign. After the campaign wearing rates fell but not to levels before the campaign. The campaign also increased seat belt use by drivers and other car occupants. The programme was school based and children were offered rewards and prizes for wearing restraints. A later study extended the experimental programme to 25 schools, where once again rewards increased seat belt use during the campaign (Roberts *et al.*, 1988). Comparison of a parent coercion and child education strategies by Bowman *et al.* (1987) revealed positive effects from education but not from coercion (see Table 15). An interesting study has recently been reported from the United States (Stuy *et al.*, 1993): this programme in child care centres was directed at professionals and aimed to change the culture of the environment at the child care centres. Parents were encouraged to sign contracts agreeing to correctly restrain their children in their cars on journeys to and from the centre and this was reinforced by classroom activities for children.

Other measures

Other devices to protect car passengers include inflating air bags and interior design of the car which have been shown to afford protection under experimental conditions (Rivara, 1985; Evans, 1991).

4. The home environment

Background

Scale of the problem

Most of the unintentional injury deaths in children under 5 take place in the home. Added to this are the very large numbers of non-fatal injuries: 647,000 children under 5 were estimated to be injured in the home in the United Kingdom in 1989 (DTI, 1992a).

The most severe home injuries and deaths are associated with fires, burns and scalds, falls, poisonings and drowning. Fires rank second as the cause of unintentional injury deaths in children under 15; around 90 children die in fires each year (Table 1). While the number of deaths occurring as a result of poisoning is relatively small (Table 1), suspected poisoning is 'expensive', requiring approximately 14,000 hospital admissions and 40,000 accident and emergency attendances each year (CAPT, 1989). Falls in the home caused 37 deaths among children in 1992 and of these about one-third died as a result of a fall from a window. Falls are also the major cause of hospital admissions and accident and emergency attendance. Choking, suffocation and strangulation also cause a significant number of deaths. In 1990 there were 41 deaths from mechanical suffocation and 17 from inhalation and ingestion, with children under 5 being at greatest risk (see Table 1).

Who is at risk?

The type of accident a child is likely to have in the home is dependent on the child's age and stage of development. Children under 5 spend most of their time in the home and are the group at highest risk, for example, 84% of poisonings occur within children's own homes. Like other injury types, boys are at greater risk than girls of death within the home (Jackson, 1977). There is also evidence that children from poorer homes are at greatest risk. Learmouth (1979) studying burn and scald accidents in Bradford found that low socio-economic group, lack of hot water and overcrowding were associated with increased risk, as was ethnic group, Asian children were over-represented amongst casualties. Alwash and McCarthy (1988) found that social disadvantage was more important than ethnicity as a determinant of accidents to children in the home.

When are children at risk?

There is a seasonal variation in risk for most injury types: more falls from windows occur during summer months as do poisonings (Spiegel, 1977). Fire injuries are greater during the winter months (Learmouth, 1979).

(Fires, burns, scalds, poisoning and suspected poisoning are also discussed separately, after 'General home injuries'. Drownings occur both within the home and outdoors and are discussed in '5. The leisure environment'.)

General home injuries

Tackling the problem of deprivation

The problem of social deprivation was addressed in a study in the USA of nurse home visitations during pregnancy and the first two years of life. The mothers in this study were poor unmarried teenagers. Homes where there had been a nurse home visitor had fewer home hazards than those where there had been no home visits (Olds *et al.*, 1994); see Table 16. The home visitation programme studied non-injury outcome measures such as child abuse and neglect and mothers' warmth and control of their children.

In an epidemiological study, Alwash and McCarthy (1987) found that common domestic accidents in West London such as falls, poisoning, cuts, burns and scalds happened when parental supervision was reduced rather than because of household hazards. Rather than urge parents to be more vigilant, they advocated tackling the underlying problem of deprivation with more financial help for families with young children and better support services (Alwash and McCarthy, 1987). We were not able to find any evaluated studies of such a strategy, though the steep social gradients in deaths from house fires (OPCS, 1988) would indicate that this would be a fruitful area for intervention.

Building regulations and home design

Sinnott (1977) and Gloag (1988) describe a range of aspects of domestic architecture which have been regulated since the 1960s to enhance home safety. Open tread stairs have been prohibited and opening distances of windows in high-rise buildings controlled. Architectural glass is a hazard for children and interior glazing in new buildings is now regulated (Department of Environment, 1991). In 1966 handrails on staircases became compulsory and steepness limited. Any direct relationship between these measures and reductions in injury rates has not been shown. There is a need for continuous close monitoring of accident reports, and field evaluations of features designed to improve the home environment, for as Sinnott remarks:

> Children are extensive users of domestic architecture; . . . [they] crawl about the floor, climb on to the window ledge, squeeze through stair

balustrades, slide down the stair hand-rail, swing on the gate, run from room to room and ride bikes inside as well as out . . . making use of their homes in ways that seem to them to be reasonable but have not apparently been foreseen by the designer.   (Sinnott, 1977)

Safe products – product design

Product redesign is an area which has shown positive effects on injury reduction. The section on burns describes the redesign of front loading washing machines to avoid devastating chest scalds in young children (Sørensen, 1976). Kraus (1985) evaluated the redesign of products associated with strangulation and suffocation – refrigerators, infant cribs and plastic bags. Over a 20-year period he recorded a significant decline in refrigerator entrapments, declining numbers of crib suffocation deaths associated with children becoming trapped between slats and the mattress, and warnings on plastic bags leading to a significant decline in suffocations. More recently, Home Accident Surveillance System (HASS) data (collected by the DTI) led to the redesign of pens to prevent child asphyxiation after inhaling caps (Mathias and Colling, 1988). Monitoring of injuries associated with specific toys, furniture and consumer goods will shed light on the design process of new products and lead to the rapid identification and withdrawal of hazardous products but this has not been formally demonstrated. Avery and Jackson (1993) provide a useful summary of children's products covered by regulations or standards in the United Kingdom.

Safety devices

While home design may make a significant contribution to future safety, this will not occur in the short term. A range of protective devices is available to improve safety within the home. The efficacy of some devices has been tested under experimental and field conditions (for example smoke detectors and child-resistant closures). Other devices have been associated with lower risks such as fireguards, stairgates, safety catches for cupboards, coiled kettle flexes, safety harnesses, safety film for interior glazing and thermostat control of tap water (DTI, 1991). However the efficacy of all these recommended devices needs further investigation. There are other devices which do not seem to be associated with significant risk reductions or may themselves introduce new threats. These devices include cooker guards and bath thermometers.

Parent and child education (see Table 16)

Campaigns and programmes aimed at raising awareness of home hazards and encouraging parents and children to behave in ways to improve safety in the home have met with varying degrees of success (Table 16). An early study by Schlesinger et al. (1966) reported no significant gains in terms of reduced injury rates from a community-wide educational campaign directed at parents of young children organised through neighbourhood groups. A later campaign (Dershewitz and

Williamson, 1977) involving personalised advice and provision of free devices led the authors to conclude that household injury control was too broad a field for health education to be effective.

Similarly, a UK study by Minchom *et al.* (1984) in Cardiff reported no significant improvements in injury rates after a campaign; however the campaign was short, penetration relatively low, and baseline and follow-up data were collected over a short period. Exhibitions on home safety such as the Department of Trade and Industry 'hazard dome' seem to have a limited effect in terms of raising awareness of hazards (DTI, 1986).

Several programmes have reported positive outcomes in terms of increased knowledge, changed attitudes, safety-enhancing behaviour and occasionally injury and mortality rates.

Dershewitz (1979) reported mixed outcomes from a programme involving the distribution of electrical socket covers and cupboard catches. The devices such as outlet covers which needed little time to install were used more than those which required more or repeated effort.

A UK intervention in Newcastle in the early 1980s (Colver *et al.*, 1982) involved a combination of a mass media campaign along with health visitor home visits. Targeted advice was given on hazard reduction and this led to 60% of the intervention group making some physical change to make their homes safer, compared with 9% of the control group (who had also been encouraged to watch the television campaign). Colver *et al.* (1982) concluded:

> Our most encouraging finding is that even most severely disadvantaged families will respond to health education if the education is appropriate.

In this intervention the purpose of the health visitor's home visit was clear and the amount of advice given was small, specific and concrete.

The studies by Colver *et al.* (1982) and Dershewitz (1979) reveal that measuring home hazards is not simple and that using hazard reduction as an 'outcome' measure is not without difficulties. The Colver study showed that families made changes to reduce hazards, the Dershewitz study showed that while families did take measures to reduce hazards the overall number of hazards present was not significantly altered by an educational campaign. A paper by Barone *et al.* (1986) describing an evaluation of an intensive intervention to reduce home hazards highlighted the imprecision of methods of auditing home hazards. Similarly, 'home hazard scores' were an 'outcome' measured by Paul *et al.* (1994). In reviewing the effectiveness of interventions it is difficult to understand the effect of reductions of hazards (in the home or outdoor environment) without clear criteria about what is included as a hazard and how precisely specific hazards relate to risk. At the moment the way that an absolute number of home hazards relates to risk or the way that any one hazard contributes to risk is unclear. It seems obvious that some hazards pose more threat than others, 'counts' of hazards may therefore be inappropriate. It is necessary to develop methods of collecting hazard data if hazard eradication or reduction is to act as a proxy measure for reduction of injury risk.

A campaign focusing on a single hazard achieved considerable success and in this study hazard reduction was related to injury rates. Spiegel and Lindaman (1977) describe a community-wide campaign involving the police, health workers and the media aimed at reducing injuries and deaths as a result of window falls in New York: 16,000 window guards were provided for 4200 families living in high-rise flats; 35% of the guards were installed by health workers. The authors reported a 50% decline in window falls in the Bronx area, 31% decrease city wide and a 35% decrease in mortality due to falls (Table 15).

Important in this campaign was the variety of approaches adopted: a mass media campaign, individual education and home inspection. Other contributory factors for its success were the range of agencies involved (community organisations, schools, clinics) and the fact that free protective devices were provided and in many cases fitted where children were at risk.

Fires, burns and scalds

Home and product design
Clearly, there is a need for building and product regulation to reduce risks from fires. Such regulations include building codes relating to kitchen design to reduce access by children to the sides of cookers (Sinnott, 1977). Many such regulations have not been evaluated. Sørensen (1976) documents changes in burn injuries occurring as a result of product re-design in the case of washing machines, coffee filters and vacuum cleaner plugs.

Laing and Bryant (1991) demonstrated a reduction in burn injuries related to children's nightwear following the introduction of legislation controlling the design of nightwear and the types of materials used in its manufacture.

These studies underline the need for good surveillance systems to identify products associated with injury, to record incidence and to follow up the results of product modification.

Smoke detectors

There have been a series of evaluations of campaigns aimed at increasing the use of smoke detectors (Table 17). Gorman *et al.* (1985) describes a campaign aiming to increase installation of fire detectors in those homes most at risk and reported that a smoke detector give-away programme involving local firefighters resulted in the distribution of 3720 free detectors and sales of detectors at cost exceeding 100,000. Of those detectors distributed free, 81% were operational 8–10 months after the campaign. A give-away campaign reported by Shaw *et al.* (1988) also demonstrated a high take-up of devices but did not record whether the detectors were installed.

A novel give-away campaign was described by Hammond and Varas (1990) where a bulk purchase scheme was combined with provision of free detectors for some families. For every smoke detector purchased one was given free to a family in a low-income neighbourhood – 6000 devices were donated and fitted as a result of this intervention.

McLoughlin *et al.* (1985) comparing smoke detector legislation across two states recorded a reduction in fatal fires (but an increase in fires) in a community where smoke detectors were required by law in all homes. However, the reduction in mortality was not large and the authors comment, using an analogy from seat belt use, that:

> unless compliance is virtually universal, the higher rates of deaths and injuries among high-risk populations are likely to mask the effectiveness of the devices for the majority of people.

Miller *et al.* (1982) suggest that a short education session at well child clinics by a paediatrician resulted in a significant increase in smoke detector installation in the intervention versus the control group homes. The study population was predominantly white and middle class, not a high-risk group. Levels of smoke detector ownership in the United States are much higher than the United Kingdom with 85% of homes having at least one smoke detector present if not operational (McCabe and Moore, 1990; National Fire Protection Association, 1990). In the United Kingdom 47% of a sample interviewed following a television advertising campaign reported that they had a smoke alarm installed (Home Office, unpublished, 1992).

Tap water temperature reduction (Table 17)

Several authors describe campaigns aimed at lowering domestic water temperatures in a bid to reduce scald injuries in children. Educational campaigns seemed to have limited but positive results. Katcher (1987) describes a community-wide campaign co-ordinated by the electricity distributing companies. Free thermometers were provided on request and there were significant reductions in water temperatures by those motivated enough to request thermometers but not by the rest of the population. Webne (1989) reported no significant results from a small-scale education campaign by a paediatrician aimed specifically at high-risk families. In a later study (Katcher *et al.*, 1989) reported some changes in water temperatures following physician counselling: water temperatures were more likely to be checked and reduced if free thermometers were provided.

Erdmann *et al.* (1991) describe the effects of legislation where new water heaters were pre-set at safe temperatures. They report reductions in scald casualties and reduced domestic water temperatures.

Two recent studies have revealed the difficulties associated with campaigns aiming to reduce tap water temperatures. Fallat and Rengers (1993) showed that a community-wide campaign resulted in knowledge gains; however, a device provided to some families as part of the intervention was found to be ineffective. The device was fitted into taps to control water temperatures. However, the majority of devices were removed as they easily became blocked and restricted water flow. A study in New Zealand (Waller *et al.*, 1993) showed that in households where hot water systems were electric it was possible for temperatures to be effectively regulated. However, when families relied on more than one form of water heating system temperature regulation/reduction was less likely to take place. These studies highlight the fact that health education messages are only likely to be effective if water heating technology is available to support them. That is, families with young children at high risk need to be able to reduce temperatures permanently by a simple, single action without causing other negative effects such as restricted water flow.

Parent and child education (Table 17)

There is no evidence that general education campaigns aimed at fire prevention have resulted in injury reduction. A large state-wide campaign in the USA, Project Burn Prevention, conducted by McLoughlin *et al.* (1982) reported knowledge gains amongst schoolchildren but no reduction in burn injury incidence or severity in the longer term. Similarly campaigns aiming at general hazard reduction (Varas *et al.*, 1988; Eckelt *et al.*, 1985) reported small increases in knowledge but no changes in behaviour. However Thomas *et al.* (1984) claim reductions in home water temperatures resulting from a short burn prevention education session at a well child clinic. An evaluation in Britain of National Fire Safety Week by McCabe and Moore (1990) reported that amongst those attending accident and emergency departments only 15% were aware of the campaign and that there was little change in attitude after the campaign.

An evaluation of a national campaign in Denmark which included public education and aimed to reduce burn injuries and hospitalisations led the authors to conclude that the campaign achieved significant injury reduction which was attributable to the intervention. However, the evaluation did not include a control group and although there were fewer burn hospitalisations in the years following the campaign it is possible that these were due to factors other than the health promotion activities.

A number of school-based burn injury prevention interventions are included in the literature and these have met with some, although limited, success (Linares and Linares, 1979; Grant et al., 1992). While a short, one-off lecture on burn hazards resulted in increases in knowledge, there was no evidence that such interventions were effective in the long term or had any effect on behaviour or injury rates. A school-based intervention described by Thompson et al. (1992) focused on teenagers as potential baby-sitters. Although the intervention appeared ineffective, older children and young adults may be an important target group as they are often responsible for the safety of younger children.

Poisoning and suspected poisoning (Table 18)

Safe packaging of drugs and household products

There is evidence from the USA (Walton, 1982; Palmisano, 1981) and the UK (Sibert et al., 1977) of the effectiveness of child resistant packaging of drugs. A study in the United States for example showed a decrease in poisonings after regulations had been introduced (McIntire et al., 1983). From January 1976 in the United Kingdom all children's aspirin and paracetamol preparations were required to have child-resistant closures or dark tinted unit packaging, and in 1981 the Pharmaceutical Society introduced a voluntary scheme to cover all medications (Ferguson et al., 1992). In the year following the 1976 Act, Sibert et al. (1977) record a 'highly significant fall in admissions for accidental aspirin poisoning'.

Even with these packaging regulations there are some problems. Many products remain unregulated, particularly some corrosive household cleaning agents. Ferguson et al. (1992), describing admissions for poisoning over a 10-year period in Oxford record that 56.4% of poisonings were due to ingestion of medicinal agents and 43.6% to other agents, in particular household products such as bleach, detergents and paint removers. A DTI report on home accident safety equipment suggests that in 1983 4 deaths might have been prevented by the presence of child-resistant closures on unregulated products (DTI, 1991).

Sibert et al. (1985) revealed that the regulation of packaging of medicinal products by a voluntary code of practice agreed between the government and the pharmaceutical industry was largely ineffective in reducing accidental poison ingestion by young children. First, many substances covered by the code of practice continued to be dispensed in non-child-resistant packaging. Further, the voluntary code related to solid-dose preparations only and a review of hospital admissions revealed that there was a steady increase in poisonings due to ingestion of liquid medications.

Nevertheless, Walton (1982) notes that 'child-proof' packaging without safe storage is far from a universal panacea as twice as many poisonings continue to occur in the USA associated with regulated compared with unregulated products.

Poison labelling

We did not find evidence of evaluation of labelling of hazardous products by manufacturers, but this seems a positive strategy which will enhance programmes aimed at parents encouraging safe storage of drugs and household products. Labelling harmful substances with poison warnings (Mr Yuk stickers) in order to deter young children from tampering with dangerous products has been demonstrated to be ineffective: young children indeed were attracted to the containers (Vernberg et al., 1984). Fortunately, this did not affect poisoning rates; there were no differences across groups supplied or not supplied with stickers (Fergusson et al., 1982). Children under 3 do not seem to be amenable to this type of educational approach (Table 18).

Safe storage of hazardous products

An evaluation of an intervention in South Africa involving the distribution of child-resistant containers for the storage of paraffin revealed that this strategy was an effective means of reducing paraffin ingestions (Krug et al., 1994). In all 20,000 specially designed paraffin containers were distributed in the intervention area. It was recognised that the storage of paraffin in intermediate containers remained a problem despite the intervention and that CRCs did not diminish the need for adequate supervision of young children and the safe storage of hazardous substances. There was also evidence that containers were insufficiently durable for everyday use. Nevertheless, this study provided evidence that many families will use a free, effective injury prevention device, and in this case reductions in injury were achieved.

Managing poisoning incidents (Table 18)

A number of studies have examined the impact of interventions which aim to reduce the injury effects after a poison ingestion. These interventions include parent education and the provision of Ipecac (an emetic for use after a non-caustic ingestion) to increase 'readiness' after a poison ingestion. The results of these studies are mixed. While Dershewitz et al. (1983) and Dershewitz and Paichel (1984) showed that counselling by health carers on poison management and the provision of free Ipecac was associated with increases in knowledge scores overall, some mothers had worse scores after receiving poison management education. Following the intervention with a group of mothers from lower socio-economic groups, 20% reported that they would administer Ipecac after a caustic ingestion without seeking advice. This intervention might therefore prove positively harmful if reported behaviour was reflected in actual behaviour. Woolf *et al.* (1987) also revealed that many parents provided with Ipecac were uncertain how to use it. Schnell and Tanz (1993) revealed increased knowledge in families receiving a mailed poison prevention package. However, these families had already experienced a poisoning incident and had contacted a poison centre. The intervention group were found to be more educated than the general population. It is possible that the intervention may have been less effective with less receptive families. Woolf *et al.* (1992) demonstrated that families receiving a mailed poison education pack reported safer storage of hazardous substances. None of the above evaluations reported any injury reductions following the interventions.

5. The leisure environment

Drowning and near drowning

The scale of the problem

In England and Wales drowning ranks third as a cause of unintentional injury in children under 15: 47 children died as a result of drowning in 1992 (Table 1). In years with warmer summers, more children die. The outcome of a submersion event is clear cut: either children tend to recover completely, regaining consciousness quickly or they suffer serious neurological sequelae or death (Spyker, 1985). The mortality to morbidity ratio is very high; Kemp and Sibert (1992) record a 48% mortality rate for children admitted to hospital after a drowning incident.

Who is at risk?

Boys over 5 years are much more likely to die as a result of drowning than girls and the gradient is even steeper for older children. The under-5 age group is the most vulnerable.

Where are children at risk?

For children under 5 years drowning is most likely to occur in or very near the home. The areas where the young child is most at risk are the bath-tub, garden ponds and domestic swimming pools. A small number of drowning deaths occur in nappy buckets or garden pails (Mann et al., 1992). For older children the area of risk moves away from the home to open inland waterways and to a lesser extent, the sea (Kemp and Sibert, 1992).

When are children at risk?

Older children (5–14) and particularly boys are most at risk during warm weather when exposure increases, this is reflected in the large difference in mortality figures in different years.

Prevention – drowning and near drowning

Parent and child education

For the youngest children, a factor associated with most deaths was the lack of adult supervision at the time of the incident. Campaigns aimed at reducing hazards and increasing parental awareness of the risks in the home, including bathroom supervision, have met some, although limited success (e.g. Colver and Pearson, 1985).

Teaching children to swim seems to offer protection from drowning injury in older children (Yamamoto *et al.*, 1992). A number of injuries occur as a result of children who are unable to swim falling into water from the bank, and some of these deaths may have been avoided if the children had been able to swim. For young children the protective value offered by swimming skills is more controversial. While a study in the USA claimed that 'water-safe' infants were less likely to need retrieving from domestic swimming pools (Whitehead, 1983) there remains the fear that teaching toddlers to swim could result in greater exposure and decreased vigilance by adults. It is interesting to note however, that in a New Zealand study toddlers did not drown while swimming, 23 of 24 children drowning in domestic pools were fully clothed and just wandered into an unfenced pool (Gardiner *et al.*, 1985).

Guarding public pools, beaches, lakes and waterways

There is evidence from Australia and the USA that beach guards are effective in reducing drowning deaths on certain beaches (Patrick *et al.*, 1979; Spyker, 1985). The small number of drowning deaths in public swimming pools in England and Wales (2 in 1988–89) also points to the value of trained guards. The ratio of near drowning deaths to deaths in public pools also suggests that prompt rescue and resuscitation by pool guards saves lives (Kemp and Sibert, 1992).

Pool design and protection – education and legislation

In Australia, New Zealand, Canada and the USA domestic pool ownership and drowning deaths are more common. Much of the evaluated research has been in pool design and pool protection. The provision of adequate fences around garden ponds and domestic swimming pools has been associated with reduced risk, particularly for the under-fives. Fences with self-locking gates restrict access to pools for wandering toddlers. Above ground rather than in-ground pools are also associated with decreased risk (Pearn and Nixon, 1977; Pitt, 1986; Barry *et al.*, 1982; Wintemute and Wright, 1990; Quan *et al.*, 1989).

The effects of pool fencing regulations in Queensland, Australia has been evaluated by Milliner *et al.* (1980); the findings indicate that pool fencing, along with effective policing and rigid enforcement, lead to decreased drowning risks. Milliner claimed that safety legislation could cut fatal and near fatal pool accidents by at least half. The study did not indicate whether it was the regulations alone or enforcement that encouraged compliance, as a neighbouring community with some regulations but weak policing was used as a control. The efficacy of pool fencing regulations has also been supported by a number of authors within the USA, Australia, New Zealand and Canada (Fergusson and Horwood, 1984; Gardiner *et al.*, 1985; Cass and Gratton-Smith, 1991; Wintemute *et al.*, 1991). These evaluations are not included in the tables as they are of more limited importance in the UK context, where pool ownership is low.

A study by Wintemute and Wright (1990) showed that pool owners were not convinced of the need for pool barriers and 61% were opposed to regulations to mandate fencing of existing pools. They appeared instead to favour first-aid training. From these figures it is clear that there is need for the climate of opinion to change in favour of barriers. Without such a change, achieved by public education, and without rigid enforcement, compliance with regulations may be low.

Play and sport injuries

Scale of the problem

Around 1.2 million children are injured outside their homes each year in parks, fairs, playgrounds, on the street, using sports facilities and in schools and nurseries (CAPT, 1989). Horse-riding accidents alone are estimated to result in 10,000 to 15,000 accident and emergency attendances and 2000 to 3000 admissions (Gloag, 1988). Although fatalities are rare, playground accidents give rise to at least 20,000 hospital attendances and many more less serious injuries (King and Ball, 1989).

Who is at risk?

Young children (0–4) are most likely to have playground accidents. Boys have more fatalities in most categories of leisure activities (Avery *et al.*, 1990) and for over-5s, boys are most at risk of being injured, especially while playing football (DTI, 1992a). For horse riding, girls aged between 10 and 14 are over-represented in the accident statistics. No information is available in the United Kingdom on the social class distribution of sporting injuries in children (Avery and Jackson, 1993).

Prevention – play and sport injuries (Table 19)

Public policy on play, leisure and transport

Changes in public policy have been advocated to make the area around children's homes safer for play. Streets frequently double as children's play areas as well as being part of the transportation network. Area-wide traffic calming schemes may make 'home zones' safer play environments for children (Preston, 1990). Greater nursery provision, more access to sports facilities and after-school clubs could potentially result in fewer casualties.

Environmental improvement

There has been little evaluation of changes in playground layout, equipment and surfacing in terms of achieving injury reduction, although all of these factors have been associated with injuries (Illingworth, 1977; DTI, 1992a). King and Ball (1989) suggest that the value of shock absorbing surfaces has never been properly evaluated under operational conditions. They also claim that the emphasis on surfaces rather than other playground features arises from a misconception about the scale and severity of head injuries, the bulk of serious injuries caused by falls involve the upper limbs.

Fisher *et al.* (1980) describe a statewide campaign in the United States targeted at local authority staff aiming to reduce playground hazards. The study revealed increases in knowledge, reductions in hazardous equipment and a claimed reduction in playground-related injuries treated at local hospitals.

A nursery playground inspection scheme in Atlanta (Sacks *et al.*, 1992) reported insignificant findings. King and Ball (1989) claim that full implementation of existing playground standards in the United Kingdom may result in injury reductions although we found there was no evidence of evaluated studies in this area.

Adult supervision and child training

Lack of adequate adult supervision has been associated with injuries in young children (King and Ball, 1989) as has lack of adequate training and motor skill development in children (Sahlin and Lereim, 1990). However, we have found no evaluated studies of training schemes for adults or children.

Protective equipment

The promotion of protective equipment for sporting activities such as rugby and horse riding is also to be encouraged (Condie *et al.*, 1993). There is a clear need for adequate injury surveillance in this area (Garraway *et al.*, 1991).

A study by Morton and Burton (1979) showed that mouth-guards were associated with reduced dental injuries in rugby players, although the authors pointed to the need to redesign the device to increase its efficacy.

6. Community-based campaigns

Background

In recent years community approaches to injury prevention have been receiving more attention. Finney *et al.* (1993) believe this is partly, 'because of concern about the tendency to focus on individual responsibility for health to the exclusion of any recognition of the structural determinants of social behaviour'. Instead of focusing on individual responsibility for health and on victim blaming, the multi-faceted nature of community-based interventions means that in certain communities interventions are so pervasive, 'that it is difficult for the citizens of the community to remain unaware and uninvolved' (Finney *et al.*, 1993).

Popay and Young have looked in detail at community-based injury interventions (both evaluated studies and continuing programmes) and believe that essential criteria are that they include involvement of local communities' networks, that they prioritise vulnerable groups and that they need to be run for at least four years (Popay and Young, 1993; Klang *et al.*, 1993). In their review, Popay and Young identify two dominant approaches in community interventions: the health planning approach and the community participation approach (Popay and Young, 1993). The former approach emphasises behavioural change and safety education; examples include Falköping, Sweden (Schelp, 1987, 1988), Motala Sweden (Klang *et al.*, 1993), Lulea, Sweden (Hammarström, 1989), Drammen, Norway (Klang *et al.*, 1993) and the Statewide Child Injury Prevention Program (SCIPP) Massachusetts, USA (Guyer *et al.*, 1989). The second approach, the community participation approach, emphasises changing the physical environment where local people shape the intervention (Popay and Young, 1993). Examples include Sollentuna district, Sweden (Bjärås, 1987), Corkerhill, Glasgow (Roberts *et al.*, 1993) and Castlemilk, Glasgow (Graham and Svanström, 1989). Of these programmes, three have published results of evaluated interventions (Falköping, SCIPP, Massachusetts and Sollentuna) and these are described in more detail below.

Within the last decade, Australia has developed considerable experience in community-based injury prevention, based on the Swedish Falköping model. The collection of the experiences of those involved in the community-based injury prevention projects in Victoria, South Australia and New South Wales is documented in *Community-based injury prevention: a practical guide* (National Safety Council of Australia, 1992). Contributors to this publication discussed their personal experience of involvement in local projects and the report consequently provides practitioners with insights on what works and does not work at a local level.

Moller from the National Injury Surveillance Unit, South Australia and a contributor to the practical guide, believes that success in community-based projects in Australia has been associated with:

- identifying the decision-making structures and methods of communities and placing injury firmly on the local agenda
- providing good information about ways of reducing injuries when opportunities arise
- setting up for a long-term involvement and transferring expertise to the community
- developing a partnership with the public and private enterprises to support the community
- being prepared to deal with those issues of interest to the community where success can be achieved and recognised.

He believes that,

> community-based injury prevention is an important process in establishing both a culture of safety and the opportunities for implementing a range of successful intervention strategies.
>
> (Moller, 1995)

Mass media campaigns on prevention of general injuries (Table 20)

In the UK two television series were produced on the prevention of general injuries in childhood. The first series of *Play It Safe* took place in the early 1980s and the second in the early 1990s. For the first series, two before-and-after studies assessed its impact on hospital admissions and accident and emergency department attendance but found no difference before and after the campaign (Williams and Sibert, 1983; Naidoo, 1984). The study by Colver *et al.* (1982) in Newcastle (described in Chapter 4) demonstrated that health visitor endorsement of the messages of the television series produced hazard reduction in houses. A small-scale evaluation of the second series showed that audience figures ranged from 8.8 to 9.6 million and there were increased reported safer behaviours (Banbury, 1992).

Evaluated community-based interventions (Table 21)

Early reports of community-based programmes which have been evaluated come from Scandinavia and the United States. Studies of programmes from Australia have been published more recently. A number of the studies are before-and-after studies without control areas (Tellnes, 1985; Robertson, 1986; Sahlin and Lereim, 1990 and Jeffs *et al.*, 1993). Only one study (Guyer *et al.*, 1989) reports a number of interventions and control communities; all the remaining studies are quasi-experimental in design, with one intervention and one control area. There are no examples of studies evaluated using a randomised controlled design.

Norwegian programmes (Tellnes, 1985; Sahlin and Lereim, 1990) Two Norwegian studies, one conducted on the islands of Voerøy and Røst and one in Trondheim claimed significant reduction in injuries as a result of prevention campaigns. But neither study had a control group and too few details are provided for the studies to be replicated elsewhere. Both studies, however, used a surveillance system as a tool in local community diagnosis and the interventions were tailored to local conditions. This is also well demonstrated by Schelp (1987) in Sweden where the results of injury surveillance in Falköping were used to stimulate local interest:

> local injury data are necessary to gain the support of local authority organisations and the population who may not believe that the problem exists in their community.

Indian health service programme, United States
(Robertson, 1986)
In the 1970s death rates from unintentional injuries were twice as high amongst native Americans as for white or black communities. In response to this, in the early 1980s the (native American) Indian Health Service began to develop community injury control programmes amongst the service units. The local programmes occurred alongside a national campaign and focused on first-aid training, smoke detectors and child restraints in cars and were initiated by inter-disciplinary committees locally. Few details are provided about the interventions which occurred, no control groups are reported and there is no evidence that the reductions in injury reported were attributable to the intervention.

The Falköping programme, Sweden (Schelp, 1987)
The intervention in Falköping stemmed from a descriptive epidemiological study of all accident cases in a defined population and defined geographical area.

As well as accurate local injury event data, the Swedish study relied on a 'reference group', drawn from a wide range of health, local authority, voluntary and commercial agencies, to coordinate and plan injury prevention activities. Within the small community of Falköping an extensive network of contacts was built up of people interested in injury prevention. Education of policymakers and health workers was a high priority and resources were produced so that, for example, district nurses had a home safety checklist to use on their home visits to parents of young children. Importance was also placed on raising public awareness and local journalists were involved in the reference group. A local shop selling child safety products was also part of the intervention and sales of these products in the intervention area were nearly twenty times those in the control area in 1982 (Schelp, 1987). Schelp found that,

> most of our accident prevention activities have been relatively easy to incorporate in different organization's existing programmes.

The Swedish study relied on one control area, Lidköping, an area of similar size and socio-demographic mix to Falköping. The comparison data concerning injury events required considerable adjustment for under-reporting in the control area, which resulted in difficulties in interpreting the results.

The Statewide Child Injury Prevention Program (SCIPP), United States (Guyer et al., 1989)

A good evaluation of a community-based child injury prevention programme is the Statewide Child Injury Prevention Program (SCIPP) in Massachusetts, USA.

In the SCIPP study nine intervention communities and five control communities were chosen from 351 potential cities and towns in Massachusetts, matching for a number of relevant variables. Five specific intervention programmes aimed at burns, poisoning, falls, suffocations and passenger road traffic accidents (RTAs) were implemented simultaneously in these communities. Outcomes were evaluated in terms of change in individual community rates of exposure to the campaign, knowledge and behaviour and incidence of injuries using surveillance data (accident and emergency attendance) for each separate programme.

An estimated 42% of households with children aged 0–5 years were exposed to one or more of the interventions over the 22 months of the intervention. Safety knowledge and profiles increased in both intervention and control communities. Households that reported participatory exposure to the interventions had higher safety knowledge and behaviour scores than those which received other exposure or no exposure to intervention activities. A significant health outcome was detected in the reduction of motor vehicle passenger injuries in the intervention communities compared to the control communities. No evidence was found in the reduction of other target injuries, although exposure to prevention messages was associated with safety behaviour for burns and poisoning. Bass *et al.*, (1991) reported on a selected sub-population of the SCIPP study and the impact of paediatric counselling on injury rates.

The authors of the SCIPP study provide a very useful critique of the study and 'the constraints of implementing "textbook" interventions in a real world setting'. They conclude:

> We cannot understate the logistics and difficulty of managing a set of complex interventions in several communities simultaneously. Our efforts to persuade local health agencies and community boards to take more of a lead role were thwarted by the unavailability of local morbidity data, a lack of financial incentives and a lack of media attention to the injury problem. (Guyer *et al.*, 1989)

Safe Block Project, Philadelphia, United States
(Schwarz *et al.*, 1993)
This is the first comprehensive injury prevention effort reported in an African-American community. The programme aimed to reduce the rates of injury occurring to residents in a poor inner city community, using community workers and recruiting black representatives from the local community. The emphasis of the programme was on the prevention of falls, fires, scalds and poisonings and on unintentional injuries and violence and included an educational programme, home visits and the provision of safety equipment. In the intervention area black representatives were recruited for 88% of the blocks, lay participation was an important element and the authors concluded that:

> we have shown that individuals with minimal formal education can be trained to co-ordinate effectively on a large-scale community-based prevention program involving community leaders, black leaders and individual families. (Schwarz *et al.*, 1993)

This method of cascade training was an interesting one and appeared most effective. There were high levels of participation in the programme: the intervention programme was carried out in 51% of the households and only 9% refused to participate.

The intervention was partially effective for those home hazards requiring minimal to moderate effort to correct: there was a distinct difference between control and intervention houses but for home hazards requiring a major effort to correct there were fewer differences.

The only minor criticisms of this study are that the census tracts selected were not randomised and that no statistical adjustments were made for an area level effect and all data are analysed as if they are individual without contamination between homes.

Safe Kids/Healthy Neighborhoods Injury Prevention Program, Harlem, United States (Davidson et al., 1994; Kuhn et al., 1994)

This programme was also targeted at a disadvantaged community in the United States. A community-based programme, it worked through a coalition to attempt to reduce outdoor injuries in children, with a secondary aim to reduce assaults to school-aged children. Specific interventions included the renovation of central Harlem playgrounds, the involvement of children and adolescents in safe supervised activities that would teach them useful skills, the provision of injury and violence prevention education and the provision of safety equipment (including bicycle helmets) at a reasonable cost. Twenty-six organisations were involved and the study demonstrated:

> the usefulness of injury surveillance both for guiding the development of a community-based and locally relevant injury prevention program and for evaluating the impact of such a program.
>
> (Davidson et al., 1994)

The incidence of injuries amongst school-aged children in the intervention area of central Harlem declined by 44% during the intervention and a significant decline was also observed in the control community of Washington Heights of 30%. In the control community both targeted and untargeted injuries declined, whereas in the intervention community the decline was specific to the targeted age group. This study had only one intervention and control area and although both were disadvantaged communities, the demographic characteristics of the two areas were different.

Illawara Safe Communities Program, Illawara, Australia (Jeffs et al., 1993)

This community-based approach to local child injury prevention was based on the Falköping model. Data from local injury surveillance were used to select priority areas for intervention which included backyard clean-ups and bicycle safety campaigns. During the period of the study the number of organisations involved increased from 13 to 26 on the task force and a total of 50 organisations participated in the child backyard safety campaign. Data from the Shell Harbour intervention area were to be compared with injury presentations from other areas in Illawara and other hospitals in New South Wales and Australia but it was not possible to do this and the authors concluded that local data had not proved useful in programme evaluation, although they were a valuable catalyst in encouraging local injury prevention activities.

The Shire of Bulla Safe Living Program, Australia

(Ozanne-Smith *et al.*, 1994)

A second example of an Australian trial of the Falköping model comes from the Shire of Bulla in Victoria. This is an example of a well-documented and carefully-evaluated study of an all-age, all-injury type prevention programme within a local community. The publication reports on the first three years of the study (1991–93) but the local council is committed for five more years (1994–98). In the initial three years, 113 preventive programmes were developed, with a particular emphasis on training professionals, environmental modification, audit and advocacy. Detailed documentation is provided by the interventions project team about the individual components of the preventive programmes (Hennessey *et al.*, 1994).

The aim of the evaluation was to investigate whether the community intervention approach was effective in preventing injuries, reducing hazards and increasing public awareness of injury prevention. This used measures of process (programme reach and community participation), measures of impact (changes in hazards and community knowledge, attitudes and behaviour) and measures of outcome (changes in injury morbidity and mortality).

A demographically matched shire, the Shire of Melton was selected as a comparison for evaluation measures and in addition comparisons were also made with the state of Victoria as a whole. A major problem has however been the considerable difference in the base level injury rates between the two shires, with the hospital admission rate for Melton over 50% higher than for Bulla.

Data from the Victoria Injury Surveillance system (VISS) have been used in the evaluation.

Process measures included programme reach and community participation. The programme was reported in local newspapers at an average level of one item per week at no cost. Over the three-year period 151 people were involved in volunteer working groups, which represented 0.5% of the Shire's population over the age of 20 years, and 300 volunteers were involved in implementing the programme (1%). Approximately 6.4% of the adult community participated in seminars and courses (for senior citizens the participation rate was 15%). A traffic safety education project, Starting out Safely, used through the state in pre-school centres, was used in 75% of the shire's pre-school centres, compared with 37% in Melton and 37% in Victoria.

Impact evaluation revealed that the Safe Living programme achieved increased levels of sales of children's safety seats and restraints, sales of smoke detectors, usage of the Early Childhood Injury Prevention Programme, wearing of helmets and training in child safety as a result of train the trainers courses. The council supported a safety audit of school playgrounds and as a result of advocacy by the Safe Living programme the schools implemented more than 50% of the recommendations of the playground safety audit.

For outcome evaluation, the number of deaths was too small to allow meaningful comparisons. Analysis of hospital admissions data showed no significant difference in injury rates between the shires of Bulla and Melton from 1987/88 to 1992/93. Length of stay in hospital was also unchanged for both shires. Vic Roads data showed a reduction in motor cycle injury in the Shire of Bulla compared with the Shire of Melton, but no significant changes for vehicle occupants, pedestrians or bicyclists. Analysis of the VISS emergency department presentations for children showed no significant difference in injury frequency for both shires. The only outcome measure which did show a change was a telephone survey which found a considerable reduction in the number of respondents who reported sustaining an injury in the previous two weeks for the Shire of Bulla relative to the Shire of Melton.

There are problems common to many community-based studies. The first is the problem of the choice of a comparison community. Here, although the Shire of Melton was matched on a range of demographic variables there was still a considerable difference in the base level injury rates between the two shires. Second, the injury rates for the Shire of Bulla were low at the start of the programme, the scope for improvement was thus much reduced. Third, in order to show a statistically significant impact on hospital admissions over the three years of the study, a 20% decrease was needed which was not realistic given the timescale and resources available. Interestingly there was a significant improvement in the intervention community of reported injury (at a lower level of severity) recorded in the telephone interviews.

Harstad Injury Prevention Study, Harstad, Norway (Ytterstad and Wasmuth, 1995; Ytterstad, 1995; Ytterstad and Sogaard, 1995) This comprehensive community-based programme to prevent unintentional injuries took place over an unusually long period (7–9 years). Injury data were used in planning local interventions and in targeting activity. A local injury prevention reference group was established to co-ordinate activities; their specific objectives included promotion of community ownership of the injury problem, diffusion of programme message and maintenance of effect.

The series of interventions in Harstad, (a small 'city' of 20,000 people north of the Arctic Circle in Norway) was based on a model developed by Schelp in Falköping and stemmed from a similar descriptive epidemiological study of all attendances at the local accident and emergency department. This injury database was used to stimulate action through a multi-disciplinary injury prevention group with attention focused on prevention of traffic injury amongst young drivers, motor cyclists, and children as pedestrian and cyclists. There was a simultaneous set of initiatives concerned with the prevention of burns in children under the age of 5. These studies are particularly remarkable for the length of follow-up received (7–9 years) but were unfortunately unable to gain any better control data than that recorded in Trondheim, a much larger city, which was 1000 km away.

The results quoted in the three papers (traffic, cyclist and pedestrians, burns), describing this work are extraordinary. With respect to traffic injuries (Ytterstad and Wasmuth, 1995), a 60% fall in attendances of children under the age of 10 is reported and a 35% fall for those between the age of 15 and 24 years. About one-third of these latter injuries were amongst drivers of automobiles and motor cycles, both groups showing substantial declines in frequency following the intervention (in the case of motor cyclists by 85%!). The interpretation of this material is made difficult by the lack of detailed comparable data from Trondheim and the known temporal changes in exposure (for instance motor cycle use in northern Norway halved during the follow-up period). The most convincing result is the 30% fall in injury rate amongst drivers aged 18 to 24 at a time when national figures for driver injury rate (aged 18–34) showed an increase for both females and males from 1980 to 1990.

Meanwhile a second paper (Ytterstad, 1995) describing in more detail the pedestrian and cyclist injuries suggested equally remarkable falls in the rates of injury for pedestrians under the age of 15 (54% reduction) and for cyclists in the same age group (31% reduction). Again there is a lack of adequate data from the control area as well as some indication that relevant exposures have decreased during the follow-up period across the whole of Norway. Nevertheless the scale of the changes observed both amongst children and young adults exceeds anything ever seen in previous injury prevention campaigns.

This must raise questions about the completeness with which data were collected in the later stages of follow-up in the intervention area. The only independent check on these rates are the 'official reports' of road traffic accidents which seemed to reflect less than one-third of the decline in traffic injuries recorded in the accident and emergency department. This is interpreted in the text as being due to an increased proportion of the hospital attenders being known to the police. An alternative explanation is that an increasing proportion of traffic injuries were actually unrecorded in the accident and emergency data system. However the measures described in the text to ensure complete recording and the fact that this was a relatively small hospital treating only some 1500 casualties per annum might indicate ideal circumstances for accurate data collection.

When the prevention of burns under the age of 5 was evaluated using the same data system (Ytterstad and Sogaard, 1995), a remarkable fall of 53% in casualty attendances was demonstrated at a time when similar attendances in Trondheim rose by nearly 10%. Although the total number of burn attendances (40) in the intervention area, was comparatively small, the findings were rendered more convincing by a parallel decrease in the severity of burns amongst the quarter of the children who were admitted to hospital.

In view of the scale of the effects which were currently being observed as a result of this intensive community-based programme, it is imperative that more detail should be given about the processes and risk prevalence changes through which the injury events have been reduced so that others can attempt to replicate these interventions in different communities.

Appendices

Appendix A. National policy initiatives

The prevention of unintentional injury is the focus of a number of governmental policy initiatives. In 1987 the Department of Transport set a target for reductions in local traffic accident casualties in Great Britain by one-third by the year 2000 (baseline average 1981–85 (Department of Transport, 1987)). Children were identified as a key target group and in 1990 a plan of action, *Children and roads: a safer way* describing how these targets could be achieved, was published (Department of Transport 1990). Two years later this was reinforced by *The health of the nation: a strategy for health in England* which identified accidents as one of its five key areas and 'the reduction of the death rate from accidents amongst children aged under 15 by at least 33% by 2005' (baseline 1990) as one of its key areas (Department of Health, 1992). In this strategy, key areas were selected because they were major public health problems, they were areas in which targets could be set and they were potentially preventable.

A major public health problem

Unintentional injury in childhood and adolescence is a major public health problem in England because:

- It is the leading cause of death in children aged between 1 and 15 years
- It is a major cause of ill health in children (Department of Health, 1992; CAPT, 1989)
- It involves the National Health Service in considerable direct costs (CAPT, 1992)
- Deaths from unintentional injury have a steeper social gradient than any other cause of death in childhood (OPCS, 1988)
- For one of the most important types of injury, child pedestrian deaths, the UK has one of the poorest records in Europe (Department of Transport, 1990).

Appendix B. The scale of the problem

Unintentional injury is a major cause of death in all developed and an increasing number of developing countries and an important cause of morbidity, permanent disability and disfigurement (Manciaux and Romer, 1991).

Costs

The annual NHS cost of unintentional injury in childhood in England and Wales has been estimated at £200 million per annum (CAPT, 1992). Other indirect costs include the social and psychological costs to families of injured children and to society. The value of preventing child road traffic accident casualties *alone* has been estimated to be £500 million per annum (calculated from Jones-Lee (1993) figures). Clearly the potential for improvement is considerable in preventing unintentional injury, deaths, disability, morbidity and the direct and indirect costs associated with these. We need to apply the knowledge of what works in injury prevention more widely and seek to improve interventions in those areas which have been more resistant to change.

Mortality

Death in childhood, after the age of one year has become a relatively rare event in the UK, and unintentional injuries are the largest single cause of death. In 1990 between the ages of 1 and 4 years injury and poisoning accounted for 24% of deaths and this rose to 37% for children aged 5–9 years and 39% for children aged 10–14 years (Woodroffe *et al.*, 1993).

Over the years unintentional injuries have been responsible for a growing proportion of all deaths in childhood and young adulthood. In the forty-year period from 1950 to 1990, in England and Wales, deaths of people aged 1 to 19 years from causes other than injury fell by nearly three-quarters; in contrast, death from injuries fell by only a quarter (Woodroffe *et al.*, 1993).

In 1992 in England and Wales 563 children under the age of 15 years died as a result of an unintentional injury (OPCS, 1994); see Table 1. Boys were twice as likely to die as girls. 40% of the children who died were under 5 years, 26% aged 5–9 years and 33% aged 10–14 years. Nearly half the children (47%) died as a result of motor vehicle traffic accidents. The next most common cause was fire and flames (15%), followed by drownings and submersions (8%), mechanical suffocation (7%) and falls (7%).

Unintentional injury death rates show considerable geographical and social variations in England and Wales. For the period 1975–84 death rates were higher in the North and West, and lower in the South and East; rates were also higher in urban than in rural areas. There was a close relationship between death rates and social deprivation. Between the highest and lowest district health authority death rates there was more than a five-fold difference (Avery *et al.*, 1990). When death rates for all injuries (intentional and unintentional) are compared with other countries, the UK fares well compared with the USA, Canada and Australia, but it has not achieved the low rates found in countries such as Sweden and the Netherlands.

Morbidity

For every child who dies, many more have non-fatal injuries. A study of childhood injuries in Newcastle in 1990 reported a death rate of 1.1 per 10,000 population, 166 per 10,000 for hospital admissions and 2149 per 10,000 for accident and emergency attendances. The Child Accident Prevention Trust estimates that approximately 120,000 children under 15 years are admitted to hospital each year and 2 million attend accident and emergency departments (CAPT, 1989). The *General Household Survey* for the period 1987 to 1989 found that 5% of children under 16 years had an accident requiring medical attention in the 3 months prior to being interviewed (OPCS, 1989, 1990, 1991).

There are few estimates of the extent to which injuries cause disabilities. Avery and Gibbs (1985) estimated that 3% of children under 15 years admitted to hospital with injury were left with a permanent disability. Barker and Power (1993) analysing a national birth cohort found that for 16- to 23-year-olds, 9% of accidents requiring admission resulted in a permanent disability.

Range of injury types and countermeasures

Unintentional injuries occur in the road, home and leisure environments and include a range of different injury types. In the road environment these include pedestrian, passenger and cyclist injuries; in the home environment there is an even greater diversity of causes of injury, i.e. fires, burns and scalds, drowning, poisoning, falls and asphyxiation and in the leisure environment drowning and sports and games injuries. For each injury type a range of countermeasures are possible; for pedestrian injuries these countermeasures include changes to the physical environment, changes in product design, increasing pedestrian visibility and changing child and adult behaviour (see Appendix C). Evaluated interventions are only available for a few of these areas.

Appendix C. Possible countermeasures to prevent pedestrian injuries

Changes to physical environment

Broad planning policies, e.g. location of schools, shopping centres, play areas

Broad transport policies, e.g. change from private to public transport, banning of lorries from certain routes

Traffic calming and management schemes (speed humps, closure of roads, banned right turns, sheltered parking bays)

Traffic speed restrictions (speed cameras, speed limits, speed humps)

Bridges and subways for busy roads

Increase in doorstep play areas

Changes in product design

Improvement in car design (to reduce the severity of injuries to pedestrians)

Increase pedestrian visibility

Promote wearing of reflective clothing

Improved street lighting

Changing child and adult behaviour

Improving children's road crossing skills

Make drivers more aware of pedestrians

Increased adult supervision of children in road environment

Appendix D. Discussion of the results

Changes since first review published

In the thirty months since the Health Education Authority published *The effectiveness of health promotion interventions: a literature review* (Towner *et al.*, 1993) there has been considerable progress in the science and art of injury prevention. There have been developments in particular in the publication of studies relating to community-based trials, bicycle helmet legislation and bicycle helmet campaigns, and to operational road safety education programmes. There are still relatively few studies in the leisure and sports area, and few new publications in drowning prevention and generally in the prevention of home injuries. In recent publications there has been more emphasis on targeting social deprivation (e.g. Schwartz *et al.*, 1993; Davidson *et al.*, 1994) and the first example of an intervention in a developing country (Krug *et al.*, 1994) documenting the distribution of paraffin storage containers.

In the period since the original review, gaps in the research evidence have narrowed in some areas (e.g. bicycle helmets) but not in others (e.g. injuries in the leisure environment).

Summary of studies contained in the review

Injuries occurring in the home, road and leisure environments encompass a wide range of causes and possible countermeasures. The published literature is not evenly spread over the different injury types; for some areas there are numerous studies reported, for example, the promotion of child safety restraints in cars and cycle helmets, but in other areas, particularly the fields of sports and leisure injuries, there have been few examples of evaluated intervention. Pedestrian injuries are notable for the fact that they account for 34% of injury deaths in childhood but there is no single countermeasure available – prevention depends on a wide range of methods.

The size and scale of studies vary enormously from the evaluation of the Harstad Injury Prevention study over a period of nine years (Ytterstad and Wasmuth, 1995; Ytterstad, 1995; and Ytterstad and Sogaard, 1995) or the evaluation of road engineering measures over a period of fifteen years (Janssen, 1991) to the evaluation of a brief school-based burn prevention programme (Thompson *et al.*, 1992). We have included 141 studies in the tables: 58% of these relate to the road environment, 31% to the home environment, 1% to the leisure environment and 8% are community-based studies. The age group most frequently targeted is the pre-school 0–4 age group (56%) followed by the 5–9 age group (43%). The young adolescent group is one where there are relatively few published evaluated studies (23%); 19% of studies targeted the general population.

Most of the interventions (87%) have some educational content and 67% of the studies included some environmental modification (in our definition this would include the recommendation of some small-scale environmental measures such as cycle helmets). Sixteen per cent of studies related to legislation.

Only 18% of studies (26) were randomised control trials (RCTs). The tables summarise the study type and other types of design used can be seen here. There are no examples of randomised controlled designs in the community-based studies. There is one RCT for experimental road safety programmes (Table 7) and two for operational road safety programmes (Table 8), two for bicycle helmet educational campaigns (Table 9), one for child restraint loan schemes (Table 13), and seven for child restraint and seat belt educational campaigns (Table 14). In the home safety area, there are six RCTs for the prevention of general home accidents (Table 16), four for the prevention of burns and scalds (Table 17) and two for the prevention of poisoning (Table 18).

The role of education, environmental measures and legislation

Unintentional injury can potentially be prevented by education, environmental modification or legislation or combinations of these measures. For some injury types a wide range of countermeasures is possible. For others such as drowning in the bath tub, environmental or legislative approaches are not possible and educational approaches are the only ones available. Health education is often viewed in injury prevention as solely concerned with individual lifestyles. Its role in influencing local and national policymakers is neglected, as is its role in underpinning both legislative and environmental change (Towner, 1995).

Combination of measures

Success is greatest when educational, environmental modification and legislative approaches come together. A good example of this is the 'Children can't fly' campaign in New York aimed at a reduction of injuries and deaths from window falls. The approaches used included individual education and mass media campaigns; free window guards were provided and in many cases fitted; and the enactment of legislation which required owners of multiple dwellings to provide window guards in apartments where children lived (Spiegel & Lindaman, 1977).

Education

Most of the education campaigns in this review have been directed at individualised behaviour change of parents and /or children. Whether education interventions are effective depends on the nature of the intervention and whether it is suited to the target group; whether methods employed are didactic or more participative; whether the number of messages is large in number or directed at one or two specific issues; the duration of the campaign; and whether other significant groups, e.g. parents, are included.

Examples of where education programmes are effective include the home safety programme in the deprived Riverside area of Newcastle where the effects of a mass media campaign were enhanced by targeted advice by health visitors during home visits. The advice given was appropriate, it was of short duration, specific and concrete and the disadvantaged families were able to respond to it because it met their immediate needs. A number of operational road safety education programmes have demonstrated that training children in a limited number of skills in real road environments or on table top models is effective in changing behaviour. Some educational programmes have shown behavioural improvement through the use of reward (e.g. Roberts, 1988). Peterson believes that 'feedback, rewards and behavioural rehearsal are extremely important to the success of educational programmes and are to be preferred to didactic and passive measures' (Peterson, 1988). In pedestrian training programmes for pre-school children when parents were actively involved they subsequently set better examples to the children they accompanied and gave more verbal instructions (van der Molen *et al.*, 1983).

There is evidence that educational campaigns in which a health professional (e.g. a paediatrician) endorses a strategy can be effective. This can be seen in encouraging the use of infant car safety restraints, smoke detectors and bicycle helmets (Bass *et al.*, 1993). Often the advice is of short duration but it is directed at a specific behaviour and the authority of the advice-giver enhances its effect. However educational contexts vary considerably. The approach used in the 'Think First' programme which was aimed at reducing brain and spinal cord injuries in youth was ineffective and possibly harmful (Wright *et al.*, 1995). This programme was a one-off lecture to a large group of students aged 11–18 years. It contained a wide range of messages and was not followed up by other curricular activities in schools.

There are relatively few examples of programmes directed at other target groups. One exception is the pedestrian safety programme in Canada where driver behaviour is targeted (Malenfant and van Houten, 1989). There is also more scope for education directed at professionals and policymakers. An example of the former is a study in the United States of a child care centre where centre staff received an educational programme which asked them to endorse and encourage the use of child safety restraints in cars by all children attending the centre (Stuy *et al.*, 1993). In the Falköping community-based study efforts were made to educate health professionals, policymakers, and local journalists about the problems of unintentional injury in the local area and to motivate their interest in the intervention (Schelp, 1987).

Environmental measures

There are a number of examples in this review of the effect of large-scale environmental measures such as area wide urban safety programmes which have reduced both bicycle and pedestrian injuries (Table 5). Environmental modification can also be of a smaller scale such as the promotion of bicycle helmets, child car restraints, the distribution of safe containers for storage of paraffin. Here education needs to be reinforced by the easy availability and the cost of the device. The Seattle bicycle helmet campaign made low-cost helmets available by a variety of subsidies. When educational campaigns encourage greater use of a device it needs to be technologically sound. A device to control water temperature for example had to be removed because it became blocked and resisted water flow (Fallat and Rengers, 1993) and child-resistant containers provided for safe storage of paraffin in a South African study were not sufficiently durable for everyday use (Krug *et al.*, 1994). In these cases the target group responded to the message but the technological device was not sufficiently robust.

Legislation and regulation

Legislation and regulation can offer a spectrum of protection from single one-off events which offer passive protection to a vulnerable recipient (e.g. design of washing machines to avoid chest scalds in young children) to those measures that offer a degree of passive protection when used correctly (e.g. child-resistant containers), and at the other extreme measures which require repetitive action (e.g. bicycle helmets or seat belts in cars). All these measures have required educational campaigns to influence public opinion and policymakers to implement legislation. For those measures requiring more repetitive action education is also necessary to maintain usage levels after legislation.

The role of healthy alliances

The bringing together of different agencies often means that a variety of different approaches can be adopted. Collaboration and networking have the potential to:

> improve and enlarge databases, promote policies based on multi-disciplinary analysis of complex injury control issues, and maximise the amount of funding available to address the problem in a co-ordinated manner. (Gallagher *et al.*, 1987)

The reference group in the Falköping community-wide study (Schelp, 1987) is a good example of a healthy alliance, developed and sustained over a number of years. The Safe Living programme in Victoria, because of the range of agencies involved, was able to develop 113 preventive programmes in the first three years (Ozanne-Smith *et al.*, 1994). One of the longest running community-based programmes which has published its evaluation has been the Harstad Injury Prevention Study from

Norway. This has taken place over a period of 7–9 years, which has allowed networks and a range of local programmes to be developed (Ytterstad et al., 1995).

The quality of the research evidence
Process
In this review it has not always been possible to assess the strength of the evidence of interventions because too few details are provided. Very often the intervention is seen as a 'black box'. There were some exceptions to this, for example, McLoughlin et al. (1982) in Project Burn Prevention, measured the programme's television exposure in hours of coverage, in the number of information booklets distributed and in teaching time devoted to it. The Shire of Bulla evaluation also provided much useful information on programme impact (Ozanne-Smith et al., 1994).

Process measures such as network analysis (tracing the progress of communication within a community) or programme exposure (determining the extent and level of exposure to the intervention, or programme acceptability either to the health promoter or to the target audience) may help in determining the more difficult questions of why a programme works in specific circumstances or localities and not in others (i.e. how transportable it is) (Nutbeam et al., 1990). This review has drawn from the world literature, but successful interventions reported from the USA or Sweden may not necessarily be applicable in Britain.

Thus there is a need for authors to report process details both to allow the strength of the evidence to be judged, and to allow others to replicate interventions which have shown positive results.

Research design
A second difficulty in judging the strength of the evidence has been where studies have no control groups. There are few studies in the area of child injury prevention which have used a randomised controlled design. In total, we reviewed 144 studies (see tables) of which 26 (18%) were randomised controlled trials (RCTs). There have been calls for increased use of RCTs in the evaluation of injury prevention and other health promotion interventions (e.g. Oakley et al., 1995; Klassen, 1995). In general, we found that more robust experimental design has been limited to single measure interventions (e.g. cycle helmets) and 'closed' systems such as schools or health centres. Single measure interventions are often chosen because it has been possible to demonstrate positive results over a limited period of time using simple experimental methods.

Occasionally weak interventions (e.g. a one-off unfocused lecture on burn prevention) were evaluated using a RCT design. In those areas where it is feasible to employ an experimental design to evaluate an intervention it is important in judging the strength of the evidence to consider also the quality of the actual intervention.

Where RCTs have been used they have mainly been to evaluate educational rather than legislative or environmental interventions. Klassen (1995) suggests that if researchers and policymakers were more 'imaginative' then it might be possible to evaluate the effect of legislation in the area of injury control using a randomised design. Given the nature of the political process this does not seem realistic. Legislative interventions are often preceded by many years of grassroots lobbying and active campaigning. This is necessary to create a climate of opinion in favour of legislative control and subsequent enforcement. Randomising states or localities to have legislation or not (e.g. mandating the use of cycle helmets) would not be feasible.

Interventions which target a number of injuries and which are aimed at dispersed groups in the population are also difficult to evaluate by RCTs. The nature of community-based interventions have led to difficulties designing studies, because of the problems of experimentally controlling so many variables. Furthermore, community-based programmes need a relatively long timescale to show effects.

Thus, while RCTs may provide strong evidence of effectiveness for some injury control measures, there are, however, injury types, injury settings and health promotion methods and settings which are not amenable to this approach. Nevertheless, it is important that in non-randomised studies suitable control groups are identified.

We have identified 22 studies in which we consider the quality of the evidence is good (see tables, marked **Good★**).

Measurement of outcomes

The analysis of effective injury prevention methods has been greatly inhibited by the lack of good outcome measures. In a number of studies which were reviewed, outcome measures were weak and there was a lack of consistency in the choice and measurement of outcome between studies which focused on the same target injury with similar target groups. This lack of consistency means that it is difficult to 'pool' findings or carry out a meta-analysis. There is a need for improved systems of data collection and this has implications for future work.

Vimpani (1989) suggests that surveillance is the key to effective control of childhood injuries. Surveillance systems can be used to target local interventions, to stimulate interest in the subject of injury prevention and to evaluate the impact of the interventions. For injury surveillance systems to be useful for evaluation purposes (and to make comparisons between, or summarise findings from, similar studies) it is necessary to have meaningful and consistent outcome measures.

Death as an outcome is too rare an event to provide information on which to target or evaluate local campaigns. Reductions in death rate could be a reflection of better medical care. It is essential to develop good quality measures of non-fatal injury. Hospital admission or attendance at emergency room/ accident and emergency departments is hardly a satisfactory measure of non-fatal injury in a community.

Where proxy measures are used for injury outcomes it is important that there is clear evidence of the association between the proxy (e.g. hazard removal, knowledge gain or behaviour change) and injury risk. In some cases, there is a quantifiable link between injury risk and a proxy measure (e.g. where changed behaviour such as wearing a seat belt is known to reduce the odds of fatal injury in a car collision). For other behaviours or hazards there is no proven link between the proxy measure and the injury outcome. For example, we do not know the odds of children falling down stairs in households with and without stair gates.

There is also a need for consistency in the way that changes in knowledge, behaviour and environments are measured. Observations of behavioural and environmental change are preferable to reported behaviour measures in that they eliminate difficulties of memory and interpretation (Finney *et al.*, 1993).

Appendix E. Methodology

1. Review of reviews: background and methodology

When the HEA literature review was published in 1993, only one extensive review had been published: this was by Pless (1993). Two additional publications extended the work of the 1993 HEA review, one examined in particular the research methodologies of the publications (Jarvis *et al.*, 1994) and the second was a more detailed annotated bibliography (Dowswell *et al.*, 1994). Since 1993 eight further reviews have been published (see Table 2) with studies of relevance to child and adolescent injury prevention. The publication by Tengs *et al.* (1995) is a more general review examining cost-effectiveness ratios for life-saving interventions. In the UK other reviews have examined the effectiveness of injury prevention interventions for two other age groups – young adults (Coleman *et al.*, 1994; Munro *et al.*, 1995) and adults aged 65 and over (Oakley and Fullerton, 1995). We consider in more detail the nine reviews summarised in Table 2.

The nine reviews have been found through searches outlined in Chapter 2 and paper copies of all have been obtained. A standardised data extraction form developed by the NHS Centre for Reviews and Dissemination has been used to extract the information from the reviews. For each publication, information has been extracted on the authors, title, date and source, and the objectives and type of the review. It continues by considering the specific interventions included in the review, the participants and outcomes assessed in the review, the study designs included and sources used to identify primary studies. We then considered how judgements of relevance and validity were made, how data were extracted from the primary studies, the number of studies included and how studies were combined. Finally the results of the review and conclusions are summarised and implications of the review discussed.

Data were extracted from the nine reviews by two reviewers (E. Towner, University of Newcastle and A. Sowden, University of York) and summarised in Table 2.

Commentary
There is very little in the injury prevention literature on cost-effectiveness of different interventions. The review by Tengs *et al.* (1995) examines 229 studies with information on 587 interventions and for each of these interventions the cost per year of life saved was estimated. A number of injury prevention interventions are included. Although containing useful comparable data and references, the information is mainly of relevance to the US context and it is not possible to estimate whether similar relative costs apply in other countries.

Three out of the nine reviews had clear selection criteria and described how studies were collected and how those included in the final review were selected (Tengs *et al.*, 1995; Bass *et al.*, 1993; and Klassen, 1995). The review by Pless (1993) was limited by its medical and mainly North American orientation but provides a very useful commentary on the studies it included. Pless makes the important point that in a number of areas of injury prevention there is compelling evidence, but that this is not always used to best advantage by practitioners. The review by Stone (1993) is a narrative one, it does not claim to be comprehensive and has a bias towards those interventions relevant to Scotland. Two reviews by Kendrick and Marsh (1994) and Mulligan *et al.* (1995) examine not only injury prevention interventions in childhood but also include young adults. Both reinforce the conclusions of Towner *et al.* (1993) and Pless (1993) for the younger age group. The second publication by Mulligan *et al.* (1995) is still in draft form, so few conclusions can be drawn from it at present. Popay and Young's (1993) review has focused in particular on community approaches to injury prevention and provides an interesting discussion about the different models employed in community-based programmes. Towner's (1994) review of childhood injury prevention was part of a wider review of general health promotion by the Dutch Centre for Health Promotion and Health Education. In this, ten studies were selected to draw out features about the range of interventions and experimental design of studies. A data extraction form developed by the Dutch centre was used for a range of health promotion areas including tobacco control, drug abuse, exercise promotion and cancer prevention.

The publication by Bass *et al.* (1993) was a systematic review which examined childhood injury prevention counselling in primary care. From 65 studies identified, 20 were selected because they were RCTs, non-randomised controlled studies or multiple time series/descriptive studies. The authors decided not to conduct a meta-analysis because of the heterogeneity of injury types, study designs and statistical methodologies employed. Bass *et al.* found that 5 out of 7 studies evaluated in a randomised controlled trial had positive effects compared with 13 out of 13 of the other studies.

Klassen's (1995) systematic review of injury prevention in children and adolescents examined educational rather than legislative interventions. His selection criteria included RCTs and non-randomised controlled studies and he conducted four systematic analyses of RCTs in home and road environments and in school-based and ambulatory care-based interventions. He calls for more RCTs in injury prevention research and recommends the formation of a trial registry.

What is notable about the nine reviews of child and adolescent injury prevention is the range of approaches adopted. Although some overlap occurs, they have their own specific objectives and focus. There are no major areas of dispute about effectiveness of different interventions; most note the lack of studies relating to specific target groups (e.g. adolescents) or to specific environments (e.g. sports and leisure).

2. Methodology used in this review
Criteria
Inclusion criteria
The main criteria for inclusion of studies in the review were that they

1. related solely or in part to the prevention of unintentional injuries

2. related solely or in part to children aged 0–14 years

3. described (a) primary prevention measures designed to prevent accidents, or (b) secondary prevention measures designed to reduce the impact of accidents

4. were studies in which an injury prevention intervention had been evaluated and some outcome measure described. Outcome measures include changes in knowledge, attitudes, reported and observed behaviour and health outcomes (changes in morbidity and mortality).

Exclusion criteria
Violence prevention studies are not included, except in those cases where they are combined with unintentional injury studies.

Identifying the literature
Literature searching and study retrieval
In conducting the 1993 review of childhood injury prevention (Towner *et al.*, 1993) we established a database of primary studies in the Department of Child Health, University of Newcastle upon Tyne. Since 1993 additional studies have been identified and added to the database. Potentially relevant studies have been identified by a variety of methods:

1. Systematic searches of electronic databases (see Appendix G for search terms used).

2. Scanning the reference lists of other literature reviews in the field (Bass *et al.*, 1993; Pless, 1993; Popay and Young, 1993; Stone, 1993; Kendrick and Marsh, 1994; Klassen, 1995; Mulligan *et al.*, 1995).

3. Scanning the reference lists of important books and articles in the field of childhood injury (e.g. National Committee for Injury Prevention and Control, 1989; Wilson *et al.*, 1991; Wols and Strange, 1993; Finney *et al.*, 1993).

4. Consultation with key informants in the field, through visits, telephone interviews and at conferences and seminars (see Appendix F).

5. Hand searching of journals, e.g. *Injury Prevention, Accident Analysis and Prevention.*

Paper copies of the reports of studies have been collected. The search strategy and search items employed are listed in Appendix G.

Extracting the data and assessing its quality

The data extraction form .

A standardised data extraction form has been developed for this study, extending from the form used in the 1993 literature review. This extraction form has been piloted and developed by the research team (see Appendix H).

Combining the findings of the publications

There is a heterogeneity of injury types, study designs and statistical methodologies which makes a numerical synthesis of results from different studies (in the form of a meta-analysis) impossible. Instead we have combined the results of the studies in a narrative review and in tabular form. The tables have been produced from the data extraction forms. The tables compiled for the 1993 review have been combined with those of the 1995 review. All the publications in the 1995 review have been independently reviewed by two researchers, while in 1993 only one researcher extracted the data and completed the tables. Time did not permit all the existing studies to be reviewed by a second researcher but an attempt has been made to supplement the information provided in the earlier tables. Where two forms were completed three members of the project team (ET, TD and GS) discussed any differences between the forms.

The tables present the following information:

1. The authors and year of publication of the paper and the country in which the study took place.

2. The injury target group, e.g. 0–4 years, 5–9 years, general population and the setting, e.g. school, primary health care, community-wide.

3. A summary of the aims and content of the intervention.

4. Whether the intervention included education, environmental modification and legislation.

5. Whether healthy alliances were involved – the range of organisations.

6. The study type, e.g. a randomised controlled trial, controlled trial without randomisation; and the sample size of the intervention and control groups.

7. The outcome measures employed – knowledge, attitudes, reported behaviour, observed behaviour, morbidity data (accident and emergency, hospital admissions, police road traffic accident data) and mortality data.

8. Summaries of the results that are considered to be the most important in relation to child safety.

9. The quality of evidence and effectiveness. An indication of the strength of the research evidence is given (see below) and how effective the intervention appears to be.

Assessing the quality of evidence of the studies
In our earlier reviews (Towner *et al.*, 1993) we found that many trials had been insufficiently controlled and that:

> More robust experimental design has been limited to single measure interventions (e.g. cycle helmets) and 'closed' systems such as schools or health centres.

There were difficulties in study design because of the problems of experimentally controlling many variables in community-based interventions. For different types of study, different criteria of quality of evidence need to be addressed. We have followed a similar format to comment on the hierarchy of evidence in the studies to that adopted in the review of interventions to reduce variations in health produced by York University's Centre for Reviews and Disseminations (CRD, 1995).

Three members of the project team (ET, TD and GS) independently assessed the quality of evidence for each of the studies listed in the tables as Good, Reasonable or Weak. We then discussed our findings and attempted to combine the information. In doing this, we felt that five categories were more useful and thus we have categorised quality as Good, Good/Reasonable, Reasonable, Reasonable/Weak and Weak. Thus a well-designed randomised controlled trial could be rated as 'Good' evidence but an RCT with a small sample size or a high attrition rate of subjects, for example, would be given a lower quality rating. The quality rating is subjective but it has been reached following discussion of three members of the research team.

Appendix F. People consulted about the review

David Lynam, Charles Downing
Gordon Harland, Nicola Christie
and Jeremy Broughton — Transport Research Laboratory

Barbara Sabey — Road Safety Consultant

Heather Ward — University College London

Sandra Hook, Martin Barnett
and Howard Chard — Road Safety Division,
Department of Transport

Peter Wilding — Directorate of Statistics,
Department of Transport

Louise Pankhurst, Michael Hayes,
Sara Levene and Hugh Jackson — Child Accident Prevention Trust

James Thomson — University of Strathclyde

Lynne Sloman — Transport 2000 London

Mayer Hillman — Policy Studies Institute, London

John Adams — University College London

Amarjit Singh and Margaret Spear — Univesity of Reading

Iain Chalmers — Cochrane Centre, Oxford

Rory Milne — Oxford Regional Health Authority

Lesley Powell — ICE Research Ergonomics,
Loughborough

John Randall — Pre-School Play Groups
Association, London

Alan Gibson — Road Safety Officer,
Newcastle upon Tyne

Pats Hollins — Road Safety Development
Officer, Devon County Council

Sean Walsh — University of Leeds

Angela Mickalide — Safe Kids, Washington, USA

John Howard and Kevin Clinton — RoSPA, Birmingham

Stephen Lawson and Michael Boyle — AA Foundation

Terry Smith — Road Safety Officer, Sheffield

Andrew Clayton — BITER, Birmingham

Deborah Sims and Wendy Broom — Transport Department,
Hertfordshire County Council

Malcolm Barrow, Yvonne Brady
and Helen Pedley — Consumer Safety Unit,
Department of Trade and Industry

Martin Ship — Fire Research

Alan Brown — Home Office

Graham Butler — Divisional Fire Officer,
Newcastle upon Tyne

Alistair MacKellar — NIPPER Programme, Perth,
Australia

James Demetre — Institute of Education, London

Alan Craft — Department of Child Health,
University of Newcastle upon Tyne

Fred Crouch

Ronni Nanton
Lother Schelp, Karin Melinder
and Gudrun Eriksson
Gunilla Bjärås

Transport Operations Research
Group, University of
Newcastle upon Tyne
Birmingham University
National Institute for Public
Health, Stockholm, Sweden
Stockholm County Council,
Sweden

Appendix G. Search strategy and search terms

Search of titles, abstracts and key words. Combination of sets A, B and C.

A.   **General + population group**
     accident*
     adolescen*
     child*
     prevent*
     safe*
     teenage*

B.   **Intervention/evaluation**
     campaign
     effective*
     evaluat*
     health education
     health promotion
     intervent*
     legislat*

C.   **Injury types etc.**
     bicycle*
     burn*
     cycle*
     drown*
     fall*
     game*
     helmet*
     home
     lacerat*
     leisure
     passenger*
     pedestrian
     play
     poison*
     restraint
     road
     safety seat
     scald*
     seat belt
     sport
     strangulation
     suffocation

Appendix H. The data extraction form

CASE NUMBER ☐☐☐   DATE OF PUBLICATION ☐☐☐☐   REVIEWER ☐☐

PUBLICATION   AUTHORS   Ozanne-Smith, J, Sherrard, J, Brumen, I A and Vulcan, P

TITLE   Community-based injury prevention evaluation report – Shire of Bulla Safe Living Program

SOURCE   Monash University Accident Research Centre

Injury type	Pedest	Cycl	Passgr	Drown	Fall	Burn/Scald	Fire	Lac	Play	Poison	Sports	Gen. home	Gen. ✔	Other

Injury setting: Home   School   Road   Leisure   Other   Community-wide ✔

Pub Type: Health   Ed/Soc Scl   Medical   Eng/Tech   Conf Abs   Unpublished   Other ✔

Place of Study: UK   USA/North America   Scan   Other Euro   Aust/NZ ✔   Other

Injury: 0–1   1–4   5–9   10–14   All children   Gen Pop ✔   Other

Target Grp

DATE & LENGTH OF PROJECT
First 3 years evaluated 1991–3

Name of Programme: Shire of Bulla

Nature and Size of Target Population Shire of Bulla
39,400 in 1991
43,900 in 1993

THE INTERVENTION
Safe Living Program

DATE & LENGTH OF INTERVENTION
1991–3 (3 years reported in this publication. Council committed for 5 more years (1994–98)

CONTENT OF INTERVENTION PROGRAMME (brief description)
In the initial three years, 113 preventive programmes developed. Emphasis in programmes on training professionals, environmental modification, audit and advocacy. Programme based on community ownership, synergistic effects of many interventions and environmental changes cumulative over time. Programmes in local primary schools, audit of school playground, 'Train the Trainer' courses, courses in first aid. Uses VISS database to inform prevention.

Aim of Programme
To establish an Australian trial of the Swedish 'Falköping' Approach

Specific objectives
To develop an all age, all injury type prevention programe, within a local community in the Shire of Bulla long-term programme, led from within the Council

Intervention by:

Health Profession – Specify
Teacher
Fire Service
Police
University researcher
Other – wide range of organisations ✓

SETTING

School
Primary Health Care
Home
Community group
Other Community-wide ✓

EDUCATION	Yes	No	Not clear
Real Life Demo			
Recommended			
1:1 Target			
Small Scale	✓		
Group	✓		
Mass media	✓		

ENVIRONMENTAL CHANGE	Yes	No	Not clear
Area-wide (specify)		✓	

(Small-scale finger-safe door jamb developed) ✓
(e.g. helmet suggested/recommended)

LEGISLATION, LOCAL REGULATIONS OR LOBBYING (specify)	Yes	No	Not clear
Legislation of footpath cycling	✓		

AGENCY COLLABORATION	Yes	No	Not clear
Schools, voluntary agencies, business and government agencies, garages, shops. Steering committee established number of working groups – e.g. Children's Safety, Schools Safety	✓		

FACTORS FOR SUCCESS OF INTERVENTION

1. Programme well resourced
2. Based on local council
3. Synergy of wide range of interlinked projects
4. Strong emphasis on environmental modification and advocacy
5. Works through community–community ownership
6. Used good source of local data in VISS

FACTORS FOR WEAKNESS OF INTERVENTION

1. Timescale – this publication is only based on 1st three years
2. Wide range of preventive prorammes developed

THE EVALUATION

Objectives of evaluation
To determine the effectiveness of the community intervention approach in preventing injuries, reducing hazards and increasing public awareness of injury prevention

POTENTIAL /STUDY/RECRUITED TARGET GROUP (ATTRITION)

Potential study group is whole community in Shire of Melton

DESCRIPTION OF EVALUATION

Evaluation to include process, impact and outcome evaluation. Detailed documentation to facilitate transfer of project principles to other areas. Comparison of baseline injuries in Bulla and comparison in Shire of Melton. 3 telephone surveys conducted survey in general practice, observation and study of cyclists for helmet wearing.

STUDY DESIGN

1. Randomised control trial
2. Control trial without randomisation
3. Before-and-after study without control
4. Other – describe
5. Time series

OUTCOMES MEASURES

Mortality Data Specify Source

Morbidity Data Specify Source

Self-report of Injury

IMPACT MEASURES

Observed Behaviour
Reported Behaviour
Attitudes
Knowledge
Other (Specify)
changes in hazards

EFFECTIVENESS OF INTERVENTION Author's conclusions

	AUTHOR	REVIEWER
Unclear/inconclusive		
Harmful		
Ineffective		
Partially effective	✔	
Effective		✔
Effective some groups		

STRENGTHS OF STUDY DESIGN & EVALUATION

(1) Uses mortality and morbidity data (VISS)

(2) Looks at process, impact and outcome measures

SIZE OF INTERVENTION GROUPS

Estimated population of Shire of Bulla

SIZE OF CONTROL GROUPS

39,400 in 1991
43,900 in1993

SELECTION OF INTERVENTION/CONTROL GROUPS, RANDOMISATION

Shire of Melton chosen as comparison community matched Shire of Bulla in demography. Both served by VISS.
Injury rates 769/100,000 in Shire of Bulla and 1177/100,000 in Shire of Melton

PROCESS MEASURES   Yes ✔   No   Not clear

Programme reach
Community participation

QUOTES RE HEALTH EDUCATION

'In practice it has been observed that some really effective prevention activities can be unpopular with policymakers, lobby groups, the public and sometimes even health professionals, while popular prevention activities are often ineffective.' (p. 74)

WEAKNESS OF STUDY DESIGN AND EVALUATION

(1) Control and intervention community have different injury rates, with intervention community having much lower rates

(2) A difference of 20% would have been needed to demonstrate a statistically significant change in admission

DISCUSSION OF RESULTS (INCLUDING QUALITATIVE RESULTS)

There is evidence to indicate achievement of 4 of the objectives of the programme.

(1) Increased community awareness of injury prevention (6.4% of adult community participated in seminars and courses, 28% of people surveyed recalled home safety package delivered to homes).

(2) Development of injury prevention strategies (113 preventive programmes developed).

(3) Hazard reduction (schools implemented <50% of recommendations of playground safety audit).

(4) Increased use of safety devices and equipment (helmets, sales of safety seats, smoke detectors).

Little evidence of achievement of objectives related to injury reduction, i.e. overall reduction in injury requiring hospital attendance on admission or reduction in bed days. At lower levels of severity the intervention community reported a considerable reduction in injury in previous 2 weeks compared to control community (telephone survey).

FUTURE IMPLICATIONS (Policy, Practice)

The true nature of the Safe Living Program can only be more fully assessed by extension of outcome evaluation over several years

OTHER COMMENTS (include reviewer's reservations and whether all objectives were met)

Very good evaluation – no reservations about judgements made

SPECIAL FEATURES OF PUBLICATION

Very well doumented programme both for the intervention and evaluation

Appendix I. The tables

In all tables Ed = Education
Env = Environmental modification
(R = Recommended, S = Supplied)
Leg = Legislation

Table 1 Deaths in childhood from unintentional injury (ICD E800–E949)[a] in England and Wales in 1992

	28 days–4 years		5–9 years		10–14 years		28 days–14 years		
	M	F	M	F	M	F	M	F	Total
Total (E800–E949)	143	85	106	43	126	60	375	188	563[a]
Motor vehicle traffic accidents (E810–E819)	34	22	63	22	81	45	178	89	267
[b]Involving collision with pedestrian (E814)	17	12	44	15	42	33	103	60	163
[b]Pedal cyclist involved in collision with MV (E813.6)	3	0	7	1	24	0	34	1	35
Other transport accidents (E800–807: 820–848)	0	0	3	2	2	5	7	7	14
Fire and flames (E890–899)	33	21	13	10	1	4	47	35	82
Drownings and submersion (E910)	23	10	8	3	3	0	34	13	47
Accidental falls (E880–888)	10	5	6	3	13	0	29	8	37
Accidental mechanical suffocation (E913)	14	6	4	0	17	0	35	6	41
Inhalation and ingestion (E911 & E912)	7	6	2	0	0	2	9	8	17
Poisoning	5	1	0	0	1	3	6	4	10

[a] ICD Codes E800–E849 are used in this table. Injuries caused by violence and self-harm are excluded. This definition is used in *The health of the nation: key area handbook on accidents* (Department of Health, 1993)
[b] Both included in motor vehicle traffic accidents

Source OPCS: *1992 Mortality Statistics, Childhood: England and Wales* (HMSO, 1994)

Table 2 (1) A review of reviews – childhood injury prevention interventions

Author, date & country	Review type & subject area	Search strategies	Selection criteria	No. studies reviewed/cited. How data extracted	How studies combined	Key results	Conclusions/comments
Bass et al. (1993) USA	Systematic review Childhood injury prevention counselling in primary care	1. MEDLINE search 2. Expert panel recommendation	1. RCTs 2. Non-randomised control studies 3. Multiple time series/descriptive	65 studies identified 20 included Each study independently reviewed by 2 people Standardised record form	Narrative review Tables Decision not to conduct meta-analysis	5/7 RCTs – positive effects 10/10 non-randomised studies – positive effects 3/3 multiple time series	Recommendation of American Academy of Pediatrics supported to include injury prevention counselling as part of routine health supervision Concentrates on counselling via primary care
Pless (1993) UK	Literature review Childhood injury prevention	1. Index Medicus from 1984 2. References cited in key texts	Not specifically stated include 1. RCTs 2. non-randomised controlled studies 3. pre- and post-test 4. time series 5. case control	Number not stated How data extracted not stated	Narrative reivew	Evidence of effectiveness for: 1. legislation for *car safety seats* 2. education & legislation for *bicycle helmets* 3. for *pedestrians* – school zone speed reductions, urban redesign, raise licensing and drinking age, lower speed limits, random breath testing *Home/Burns* Education & legislation for smoke detectors *Falls* – window guards, stair guards *Poisonings* – enforcement of child-resistant containers	There is compelling evidence in a number of areas but the evidence is not being used to best advantage by practitioners Some imitations because of its medical and North American orientation but useful commentary

Table 2 (2) A review of reviews – childhood injury prevention interventions

Author, date & country	Review type & subject area	Search strategies	Selection criteria	No. studies reviewed/cited How data extracted	How studies combined	Key results	Conclusions/comments
Pless (continued)						*Drowning* – pool fencing regulation, swimming lessons and life saving *Leisure* – regulate and enforce playground standards *Athletics* – safety equipment regulations	
Popay and Young (1993) UK	Literature review Childhood injury prevention particularly community approaches	1. DHSS 2. MEDLINE 3. Social Science Citation Index 4. Sociological Abstracts	1. Evaluated 2. Non-evaluated studies	Number not stated overall but 11 community-wide studies included How data extracted not stated	Narrative review Tables	1. Community-wide approach can be effective, leading to 30% reduction in accidents in other settings: 2. evidence is of poor quality and often contradictory 3. general campaigns ineffective 4. educational campaigns linked to practical follow-up advice sessions more impact	1. Lack of evaluation of generic community interventions 2. Need for further evaluation in this area Review focuses particularly on community approaches to injury prevention

Table 2 (3) A review of reviews – childhood injury prevention interventions

Author, date & country	Review type & subject area	Search strategies	Selection criteria	No. studies reviewed/cited How data extracted	How studies combined	Key results	Conclusions/comments
Stone (1993) UK	Literature review Accident prevention (special reference to Scotland)	1. MEDLINE from 1980 2. Search of library catalogues 3. Discussion with statutory and voluntary agencies	Not clear	Number not stated How data extracted not stated	Narrative review	1. Few evaluation studies and those available are methodologically weak 2. Major obstacle – lack of local surveillance system 3. Environmental measures – window guards, smoke detectors, water thermostats more effective than educational measures 4. Legislation on car seats and bicycle helmets effective 5. Few interventions in leisure environment 6. Few interventions occurred in Scotland	1. Much work on injury prevention remains to be done 2. Priorities to develop good practice in local injury prevention and evaluation of environmental community-wide interventions Review does not claim to be comprehensive and has strong bias towards Scotland
Tengs et al. (1995) USA	Cost-effectiveness ratios Life-saving interventions (primary, secondary and tertiary prevention)	1. On-line databases 2. Bibliographies of textbooks and review articles 3. Conference abstract manuscripts	1. Written in English 2. Information relevant to US context 3. Contained information on cost per year of life	1200 documents identified 229 met selection criteria 229 studies with information on 587 interventions	Cost-effectiveness estimates calculated in US dollars Narrative review Tables	1. for 587 interventions Cost/year life estimated Number of injury prevention interventions included – mandatory seat belt use, child restraint law Flammability standards for children's sleepwear 2. More costly to save a year of life through averting injury than through medicine	Enormous variations occur in costs of saving a life Results limited by accuracy of data and assumptions upon which original analyses made

Table 2 (4) A review of reviews – childhood injury prevention interventions

Author, date & country	Review type & subject area	Search strategies	Selection criteria	No. studies reviewed/cited / How data extracted	How studies combined	Key results	Conclusions/comments
Tengs *et al.* *(continued)*						3. More costly to save a year of life through toxin control than through averting injury	
Towner (1994) UK	Literature review Childhood injury prevention (part of wider review of effectiveness of general health promotion)	Database from 4 sources 1. Bibliographical searches e.g. MEDLINE, DHS database, Inst. Road Research Directory 2. Library searches of HEA, CAPT 3. Existing reviews hand searched 4. Consultation with key informants	1. Interventions using education as main strategy 2. Clear description of intervention and objectives 3. one pre- and post-measurement	10 studies selected to draw out features about the range of interventions and experimental design of studies Standardised questionnaire used to extract information	Narrative review Tables	Effective programmes include 1. use of local surveillance systems 2. range of educational, environmental and legislative approaches 3. educational campaigns directed at specific messages rather than advice	Future research needed: 1. to identify good outcome measures 2. to include more behavioural techniques 3. to develop more process measures Not a comprehensive review but studies selected to illustrate a variety of points
Kendrick and Marsh (1994)	Literature review Childhood and young people injury prevention	1. MEDLINE 2. ASSIA 3. DHSS 4. OHSI databases Review period 1977–1993	Not separately stated but text includes 1. RCTs 2. non-randomised controlled trials 3. quasi-experimental studies 4. time series	Number not stated Not clear how data extracted	Narrative review	For 0–15 evidence of effectiveness for: *Home* Smoke detectors, window guards, CRCs, legislation for overhead staircases and architectural glass *Road* Seat belt use, child car safety seats, cycle helmets, community-wide traffic schemes	1. Greatest success when educational, environmental and legislative measures combined 2. Educational approaches alone can change knowledge, attitudes and behaviours but less evidence for reducing injuries

Table 2 (5) A review of reviews – childhood injury prevention interventions

Author, date & country	Review type & subject area	Search strategies	Selection criteria	No. studies reviewed/cited How data extracted	How studies combined	Key results	Conclusions/comments
Kendrick and Marsh (continued)						*Sports* Lifeguards, pool fencing, training in sports, hard hats for horse riding, protective equipment	
Klassen (1995) Canada	Systematic review, Injury prevention in children and adolescents Home and road environments School and primary health care interventions Educational rather than legislation	1. MEDLINE 2. ERIC 3. Other relevant articles 4. Writing to authors 5. Hand searching of 3 journals	2 observers selected studies 1. RCTs 2. non-randomised controlled studies	535 studies identified by 2 reviewers 103 met inclusion criteria 7 RCTs for home injuries 14 RCTs for road injuries School-based – 4 RCTs Ambulatory care – 10 RCTs One reviewer extracted data and second checked for accuracy	Narrative review Tables 4 systematic reviews 1. RCTs in home environment 2. RCTs in road environment 3. School-based interventions 4. Ambulatory care interventions	1. Poor study quality is a fundamental problem 2. Some evidence that educational interventions work in school and ambulatory settings 3. Adolescent age group – evidence for effectiveness lacking	1. Formation of a trial registry recommended 2. Need for more RCTs in injury prevention 3. Large sample sizes needed to detect changes in injury rates 4. Multicentre collaborative research recommended Good systematic review but only looks at educational settings
Mulligan *et al.* (1995) UK	Injury prevention in children and young people Home, road, leisure and sports and workplace settings examined	From 1982 to 1994 1. MEDLINE 2. HEALTH PLAN 3. DATA STAR 4. DHSS 5. Article references hand searched	Levels of evidence examined 1. effective conclusive evidence 2. of theoretical benefit but subject to limited or conflicting evidence 3. little or no effectiveness	Number not stated Not clear how data extracted	Tables	1. Greatest success in injury prevention when combination of approaches used collaboration of different agencies 2. Isolated and untargeted education ineffective but education effective if targeted or combined with other approaches	Draft version no overall conclusions

Table 3 Child casualties in road accidents in England and Wales in 1992

	0–4			5–9			10–14			Total		
	Male	Female	Total	Male	Female	Total	Male	Female	Total	Male	Female	Total
Pedestrian Fatal	22	10	32	32	12	44	37	35	72	91	57	148
Seriously injured	425	216	641	1027	498	1525	1007	730	1737	2459	1444	3903
Slightly injured	1321	760	2081	3273	1709	4982	3206	2559	5765	7800	5028	12828
Total	**1768**	**986**	**2754**	**4332**	**2219**	**6551**	**4250**	**3324**	**7574**	**10350**	**6529**	**16879**
Pedal cyclist Fatal	2	0	2	8	0	8	21	0	21	31	0	31
Seriously injured	21	0	21	240	32	272	532	109	641	793	141	934
Slightly injured	94	19	113	1235	260	1495	2972	696	3668	4301	975	5276
Total	**117**	**19**	**136**	**1483**	**292**	**1775**	**3525**	**805**	**4330**	**5125**	**1116**	**6241**
Car occupant Fatal	10	7	17	9	4	13	5	10	15	24	21	45
Seriously injured	131	132	263	171	163	334	208	211	419	510	506	1016
Slightly injured	1523	1471	2994	1794	2014	3808	1688	2259	3947	5005	5744	10749
Total	**1664**	**1610**	**3274**	**1974**	**2181**	**4155**	**1901**	**2480**	**4381**	**5539**	**6271**	**11810**
Other vehicle[a] Fatal	2	1	3	1	0	1	0	4	4	3	5	8
Seriously injured	12	10	22	33	8	41	68	33	101	113	51	164
Slightly injured	196	182	378	200	201	401	415	378	793	811	761	1572
Total	**210**	**193**	**403**	**234**	**209**	**443**	**483**	**415**	**896**	**927**	**817**	**1744**

[a]Includes motorcycle, bus or coach, LGV, HGV and vehicle type unknown

Source: P Wilding, Directorate of Statistics, Department of Transport

Table 4 The road environment – transport policies

Author, date & country	Injury target group & setting	Aims & content of intervention	Ed	Env	Leg	Healthy alliances	Study type & sample size	Outcome measures	Key results	Quality of evidence and effectiveness
Boxall (1988) UK	4–11 Road policy	Following difficulties in filling vacancies for crossing patrols at schools, accidents compared at staffed and different types of unstaffed sites near schools		✔		No	Controlled trial without randomisation I = 69 stopped sites C1 = 15 C2 = 18 C3 = 10 (C1 = sites where criteria were not met for crossing) C2 = sites where staff could not be recruited C3 = other sites)	Road traffic accidents at or near sites	At 69 staffed sites 8 accidents (1 reported by crossing patrol) in 5-year period Reduced accident rates were reported for staffed sites	Evidence of **Reasonable** quality *Effective* Provision of crossing patrollers gave lowest accident rates

Table 5 (1) The road environment – area-wide engineering measures

Author, date & country	Injury target group & setting	Aims & content of intervention	Ed	Env	Leg	Healthy alliances	Study type & sample size	Outcome measures	Key results	Quality of evidence and effectiveness
Engel (1982) Denmark	General population Community-wide in city of Østerbro	Package of 25 engineering countermeasures		✓		No	Before-and-after (control accidents not areas)	Accidental injuries	Estimated reduction of 15% in accidental injuries, 10 of countermeasures had significant effect	Evidence of **Reasonable** quality *Partially effective*
Jörgensen (1985) Denmark	General population Community-wide	28 cities in Denmark involved in social safety measures		✓		No	Controlled trial without randomisation	Accidental injuries	Reduction of accidents between cyclists and cars. Increase in accidents between cyclists and pedestrians	Evidence of **Good/Reasonable** quality *Effective for some groups*
Walker & Gardner (1989) Nelson	General population children	Urban safety project Package of engineering measures individually targeted to local conditions		✓		Highway & transport committee, police, bus companies, public consultation	Controlled study Before-and-after observations in each of 5 cities Intervention area and control area selected	Police Stats 19 data Road traffic casualties	Accident reduction 7% Accident reduction 14%	Evidence of **Good*** quality *Effective* Overall reduction of 13% in accidents for all types of injury and all ages
Walker & McFetridge (1989) Bradford	General population	Measures to redistribute traffic and improve safety of individual roads			✓					Reduction in slight accidents more than in fatal and serious accidents
Ward et al. (1989) Reading	General population								Initially, increase in accidents, modifications made Accident reduction 4–15%	

TABLE 5 (2) The road environment – area-wide engineering measures

Author, date & country	Injury target group & setting	Aims & content of intervention	Ed	Env	Leg	Healthy alliances	Study type & sample size	Outcome measures	Key results	Quality of evidence and effectiveness
Ward et al. (1989) Sheffield	General population			✔					Accident reduction 20–32% Pedestrian injuries reduced	
Ward et al. (1989) Bristol	General population comunity-wide			✔					Estimated reduction 10–25%	
Doldissen & Draeger (1990) Germany	General population Community-wide	Package of engineering measures Encouragement of cycling, walking, public transport in Buxtehude	✔	✔		Inter-ministry collaboration	Before-and-after study	Accidental injuries	Reduction of 46% in pedestrian injuries. Increase of 32% in cycle injuries (40% increase in cycle traffic: cyclist accident risk has been reduced)	Evidence of **Weak** quality *Partially effective* More cyclists encouraged to cycle
Nielsen (1990) Denmark	Children 9–15 years Schools Community-wide	Collaborative work with schools, parents, engineering measures introduced in Odense	✔	✔		Schools, parents associations, police	Before-and-after study	Accidental injury, satisfaction	Accidents reduced by 85% Accidents less severe School and parental satisfaction	Evidence of **Weak** quality *Effective*

TABLE 5 (3) The road environment – area-wide engineering measures

Author, date & country	Injury target group & setting	Aims & content of intervention	Ed	Env	Leg	Healthy alliances	Study type & sample size	Outcome measures	Key results	Quality of evidence and effectiveness
Janssen (1991) Netherlands	General population Community-wide	Package of engineering measures, 3 options of combined measures (1) very simple measures to exclude through traffic (2) more extensive measures to exclude most local traffic and reduce speeds (3) Woonerf model complete reconstruction of pedestrian priority areas		✔			Controlled trial without randomisation	Accidental injuries (data collected over 15-year period)	Reduction of 25% in accidental injuries. Most expensive option on Woonerf model (3) not as effective as speed limiting option (2)	Evidence of **Good/ Reasonable** quality *Effective* but most complex package was not the most successful at reducing injuries

Table 6 The road environment – road safety education – drivers

Author, date & country	Injury target group & setting	Aims & content of intervention	Ed	Env	Leg	Healthy alliances	Study type & sample size	Outcome measures	Key results	Quality of evidence and effectiveness
Malenfant & Van Houten (1989) Canada	General Population Community-wide Schools	'Courtesy Promotes Safety' programme Multifaceted pedestrian safety programme to encourage drivers to yield to pedestrians at cross-walks School training & public education, engineering measures & police enforcement Both drivers and pedestrians targeted	✓	✓	✓	Schools Police Traffic Authors Media	Before-and-after study without control in 3 cities I_1 = 95,000 total pop I_2 = 40,000 total pop I_3 = 65,000 total pop	Morbidity data Police accident data Observed behaviour	Motorists yielding to pedestrians increased. I_1 54% 81% I_2 9% 68% I_3 44% 71% Claimed small reductions in pedestrians struck by car in I_1 & I_2 Programme well received Costs relatively inexpensive	Evidence of **Reasonable** quality *Partially effective* Evidence of improved driver & pedestrian behaviour but limited effect on pedestrian casualties

Table 7 (1) The road environment – road safety education – experimental programmes

Author, date & country	Injury target group & setting	Aims & content of intervention	Ed	Env	Leg	Healthy alliances	Study type & sample size	Outcome measures	Key results	Quality of evidence and effectiveness
Yeaton & Bailey (1978) USA	5–9 years School	One-to-one real-life demonstration to teach 6 street crossing skills Training by school crossing patrols	✓			Crossing patrol, schools	Before-and-after study I = 24 2 schools	Observed behaviour	Skills improved from 48 to 97% (school 1) and 21 to 86% (school 2) Maintained at 1 year	Evidence of **weak** quality *Effective* Observations based as children crossing roads individually through they often crossed in groups
Young and Lee (1987) UK	5 years School	One-to-one training in in timing skills to cross road on 'simulated road' 2 groups – group 1 trained in crossing single lane followed by 2 lanes Group 2 – 2 way crossing	✓			No	Before-and-after study (comparison of 2 training methods) I_1 = 23 I_2 = 15	Observed behaviour on pretend road	Improved efficiency in making use of gaps. Skills maintained at 3 weeks	Evidence of **Reasonable** quality *Partially effective* 'Simulated' roads used
van Schagen (1988) Netherlands	5–9 years	One-to-one training at the road side	✓			No	Controlled trial without randomisation I = 26 C = 47	Reported behaviour	Improvements in skills of children reported	Evidence of **Good*** quality *Partially effective* Crossing decisions recorded on computer, no real-life crossings

Table 7 (2) The road environment – road safety education – experimental programmes

Author, date & country	Injury target group & setting	Aims & content of intervention	Ed	Env	Leg	Healthy alliances	Study type & sample size	Outcome measures	Key results	Quality of evidence and effectiveness
Nishioka et al. (1991) Japan	4–6 years School	Group training aimed at dashing out behaviour 2 groups with different degrees of verbal instructions on simulated road	✔			No	Before-and-after study with 2 group comparison $I_1 = 85$ $I_2 = 79$	Reported behaviour	Improvements in behaviour dependent on level of training. 40% of children showed unsafe behaviour *after* training	Evidence of **Reasonable** quality *Partially effective* No observations in real road environment
Rivara et al. (1991) USA	5–9 years School	One-to-one real-life demonstration of 4 crossing behaviours, walking, stopping, looking and keep looking One component of community-wide programme of road crossing skills	✔			No	Before-and-after study $I = 230$	Observed behaviour	Significant improvement in looking and keep looking No effect on walking and stopping	Evidence of **Reasonable** quality *Partially effective* Unobtrusive observations in real road environment
Ampofo-Boateng et al. (1992) UK	5–11 years School	Group training to find safe places to cross – comparison of roadside and classroom training	✔			No with randomly	Before-and-after study selected control group	Reported behaviour equally effective.	Roadside and classroom training *Partially effective* More safe routes selected by trained groups. Deterioration in short term but trained groups still better than untrained groups after 2 months	Evidence of **Good**/ **Reasonable** quality

Table 7 (3) The road environment – road safety education – experimental programmes

Author, date & country	Injury target group & setting	Aims & content of intervention	Ed	Env	Leg	Healthy alliances	Study type & sample size	Outcome measures	Key results	Quality of evidence and effectiveness
Demetre *et al.* (1992) UK	5 years School	Training in timing skills to cross pretend road	✔			No	Before-and-after study	Observed behaviour on pretend road	Improved effectiveness in making use of gaps	Evidence of **Reasonable** quality *Partially effective*
Thomson *et al.* (1992) UK	5 years School	Group training in skills to find safe places to cross. Comparison of roadside and classroom training using a table top model Six half-hour long sessions	✔			No	Randomised controlled trial $I_1 = 10$ $I_2 = 10$ $C = 10$	Reported behaviour and knowledge	No difference in 2 training methods Roadside and classroom training resulted in significant improvements Increase from 10 to 30% in safe crossing skills retained over 2-month period	Evidence of **Reasonable** quality *Partially effective* No observations of children in real road environments

Table 8 (1) The road environment – road safety education operational programmes (traffic clubs)

Author, date & country	Injury target group & setting	Aims & content of intervention	Ed	Env	Leg	Healthy alliances	Study type & sample size	Outcome measures	Key results	Quality of evidence and effectiveness
Schioldborg (1976) Norway	Pre-school children Home	Children's Traffic Club Practical intervention and training by parents Children enrolled on third birthday and materials distributed every 6 months	✔			Parents	Controlled trial without randomisation	Injury rates Observed behaviour	No effect on traffic behaviour. Reported 20% reduction in casualty rates and 40% reduction in Oslo	Evidence of **Reasonable** quality *Partially effective*
Downing et al. (1981) UK	3–3½ years Home	Children's Traffic Club Booklet produced for parents to assist in teaching young children road safety and encourage appropriate levels of supervision	✔			No	I=1560 Randomised controlled trial	Reported behaviour Knowledge	Small increase in knowledge in parents who received booklets Mothers receiving booklets more likely to teach children about road safety (70%) compared to 50% in last 8 weeks Materials well received by parents and children	Evidence of **Good*** quality *Partially effective* No effect on behaviour
Antaki et al. (1986) UK	5 years School	School-based Road safety education using Tufty materials	✔			Schools, road safety officers	Controlled trial without randomisation I = 13 schools C = 18 schools	Knowledge	All children improved test scores over the 6 months' period, however children exposed to Tufty materials performed no better at the post test than non-intervention group	Evidence of **Good*** quality *Ineffective/ inconclusive*

Table 8 (2) The road environment – road safety education operational programmes (traffic clubs)

Author, date & country	Injury target group & setting	Aims & content of intervention	Ed	Env	Leg	Healthy alliances	Study type & sample size	Outcome measures	Key results	Quality of evidence and effectiveness
Tucker (1992) UK	3–5 years Home	Children's Traffic Club Parents of pre-school children invited to join traffic club Road safety knowledge and behaviour taught by parents	✓			No	Controlled trial without randomisation I = 7 counties in Eastern Region C = 6 counties	Knowledge Reported behaviour Awareness	Club membership at 49% of relevant age group. Claims some improvements in reported behaviour amongst traffic club members – 16% reported stopping at kerb compared to 4% of non-members	Evidence of **Good**[*] quality *Partially effective*
West et al. (1993) UK	3–5 years Home	Children's Traffic Club All intervention children invited to join club on 3rd birthday. Parents received mailed age-appropriate booklets to teach road safety knowledge and behaviour and encourage supervision	✓			No	Controlled trial without randomisation Survey 1 I = 459 C = 573 respondents Survey 2 I = 799 C = 802 respondents	Reported behaviour Attitudes Knowledge	Traffic Club seemed to have little effect on children's knowledge or reported behaviour, except for reducing incidence of children running on ahead of parents when out walking. No effect on whether children crossed road alone, played unsupervised in street or rode bicycles unsupervised Materials favourably received.	Evidence of **Good**[*] quality *Partially effective/ inconclusive* Traffic Club members may have over-reported safer behaviour.

Table 8 (3) The road environment – road safety education operational programmes (traffic clubs)

Author, date & country	Injury target group & setting	Aims & content of intervention	Ed	Env	Leg	Healthy alliances	Study type & sample size	Outcome measures	Key results	Quality of evidence and effectiveness
Gregersen & Nolen (1994) Sweden	3–7 years Home Schools	Children's Traffic Club Parents received mailed age-approp. booklets. Received 9 packages in total at 6-month intervals. To teach road safety knowledge & behaviour & to increase parents knowledge of children's limited ability in traffic Also used in pre-schools	✔			Schools Pre-schools Parents Nat Soc. Road Safety	Controlled trial without randomisation I=1500 C=671	Reported behaviour Self-report of injury	Members reported significantly higher traffic accident risk. I used bicycle helmets more than C. Use of child restraints in cars high in both groups Reported exposure to traffic environment greater in C than in I	Evidence of **Reasonable** *Ineffective, possibly harmful* Results possibly due to reporting bias by club members
Bryan-Brown (1994) UK	3½–4 years Home	Children's Traffic Club All intervention children invited to join club on 3rd birthday. Parents receive mailed age-appropriate booklets to teach road safety know-ledge & behaviour and encourage supervision	✔			No	Controlled trial without randomisation Survey 1 I = 500 C = 500 Survey 2 I = 200	Reported behaviour Attitudes Knowledge of children and carers	Club membership varied from 50% to 37% in different counties. Members reported a reduction in children playing in streets, an increase in carers holding child's hand on pavement, and in promotion of children stopping when told and increase in road safety education Non-members watched local safety programmes on TV with child more	Evidence of **Good*** quality *Partially effective*

Table 8 (4) The road environment – road safety education operational programmes (traffic clubs)

Author, date & country	Injury target group & setting	Aims & content of intervention	Ed	Env	Leg	Healthy alliances	Study type & sample size	Outcome measures	Key results	Quality of evidence and effectiveness
Bryan-Brown (1995) UK	3–5 years Home	Children's Traffic Club All intervention children invited to join club on 3rd birthday. Parents receive mailed age-appropriate booklets to teach road safety knowledge and behaviour and encourage supervision	✔			No	Controlled trial without randomisation	Mortality data Morbidity data (Police Stats 19)	In 2 years of free scheme 81,000 children in I area joined club (50% population 3-year-olds) 20% reduction in casualties involving children emerging from behind a vehicle Other reductions between I & C areas observed but not statistically significant	Evidence of **Good*** quality *Partially effective* May be some consequences of other car safety campaigns

Table 8 (5) The road environment – road safety education – other operational programmes

Author, date & country	Injury target group & setting	Aims & content of intervention	Ed	Env	Leg	Healthy alliances	Study type & sample size	Outcome measures	Key results	Quality of evidence and effectiveness
Preusser et al. (1984) USA	4–14 years School	Willy Whistle Campaign Mass media and school campaign to reduce mid-block dart and dash accidents in 3 cities	✔			TV, schools Mass media	Controlled trial without randomisation various studies 8,000 observations	Observed behaviour Pedestrian accident reports (state records)	Observed behaviour showed some improvements e.g. search increased from 22% before to 30% after the intervention in Los Angeles Dart and dash accidents reduced by 31% in 4-, 5- and 6-year olds	Evidence of **Reasonable** quality *Effective*
Preusser et al. (1988) USA	9–12 years School	*'And Keep Looking'* – Film to teach pedestrian skills to older children in schools Media campaign	✔			Schools Mass media	Controlled trial without randomisation several studies	Knowledge Observed behaviour Accident reports	An improvement in knowledge and behaviour scores was reported There is also a claim that there was a 20% reduction in accidents for the target age group after the campaign	Evidence of **Reasonable** quality *Partially effective*
Harland & Tucker (1994) UK	5–8 years School	'Let's decide – Walk Wise' Programme Pedestrian training resource used in primary schools integrated into the curriculum. Six practical sessions in local road environment and classroom training using table-top models (Ampofo -Boateng et al., 1992)Training by teachers and parent volunteers	✔			Teachers Parents Road safety officers Researchers	Controlled trial without randomisation I= 8 schools (sample 127 tested) C= 3 schools (sample 69 tested)	Observed behaviour Knowledge Attitudes	In I schools more children selected safe routes on table-top models. Differences were more marked in more 'compliant' *v.* less 'compliant' schools. In the highly compliant schools the proportion of safe crossing places selected by pupils increased from 0.56 to 0.84. Materials well received by teachers	Evidence of **Good/ Reasonable** quality *Partially effective* Observations based on table-top model and not behaviour in the real road environment

TABLE 8 (6) The road environment – road safety education – other operational programmes

Author, date & country	Injury target group & setting	Aims & content of intervention	Ed	Env	Leg	Healthy alliances	Study type & sample size	Outcome measures	Key results	Quality of evidence and effectiveness
Penna and Lambert (1994) Australia	8–10 years School Community-wide	Streets Ahead School-based traffic safety education programme. Integration of curricular activities and real traffic experience Delivered by teachers	✔			Schools Researchers Traffic authority	Controlled trial without randomisation I = 649 C=539 9 schools in each	Observed behaviour Reported behaviour Attitudes Knowledge	Small improvement in attitude scores in 8 of 9 I schools compared to C. 4 of 9 I schools showed increased knowledge scores compared to C. No change in children's crossing behaviour. Two schools showed improved behaviour 10–15% (These schools practised crossing behaviour at 'real sites' to greater extent)	Evidence of **Good*** quality *Partially effective* Resource well received (Observed real crossing behaviour by video)
Tziotis (1994) Australia	5–12 years School Community-wide	Safe Routes to School School-based integrated package of engineering and educational measures, e.g. erection of pedestrian fences, installation of school crossings. Measures were response to problems identified by community	✔	✔	✔	Schools Parents Local authority Local residents Vic Roads project team	Controlled trial without randomisation I= 8 cities C = Melbourne metropolitan areas	Morbidity data Police casualty data	Small amount of safety benefits provided for primary-school children, especially those riding bikes	Evidence of **Reasonable** quality *Inconclusive* (small-scale study, author recommends further evaluation using methods similar to Penna & Lambert, 1994)

TABLE 8 (7) The road environment – road safety education – other operational programmes

Author, date & country	Injury target group & setting	Aims & content of intervention	Ed	Env	Leg	Healthy alliances	Study type & sample size	Outcome measures	Key results	Quality of evidence and effectiveness
Van Schagen & Brookhuis (1994) Netherlands	8–9 years School	Training methods to teach young cyclists to behave correctly in interaction with other traffic at intersections I_1 theory & traffic training ground instruction I_2 training ground instruction	✔			No	Randomised controlled trial $I_1 = 17$ $I_2 = 17$ $C = 15$	Observed behaviour Knowledge	Neither of 2 training approaches successful in improving priority decisions of young cyclists but some positive effect on signalling and visual search behaviour	Evidence of **Good/ Reasonable** quality *Partially effective/ inconclusive*
Wright et al. (1995) USA	11–18 years School	Think First Programme School-based educational programme One-hour lecture to large group on prevention of head and spinal injuries	✔			No	Controlled trial without randomisation $I = 6$ schools $C = 1$ school	Observed behaviour Reported behaviour Attitudes Knowledge	No significant changes in attitude scores in I compared to C. Increases in knowledge in younger pupils in I but not in older pupils. Students reported more unsafe behaviours after intervention No impact on observed seatbelt and helmet use	Evidence of **Reasonable** quality *Ineffective/ Possibly harmful* Short one-off intervention with attempt to measure multiple outcomes

Table 9 (1) The road environment – bicycle helmet educational campaigns

Author, date & country	Injury target group & setting	Aims & content of intervention	Ed	Env	Leg	Healthy alliances	Study type & sample size	Outcome measures	Key results	Quality of evidence and effectiveness
Wood et al. (1988) Australia	General population Community-wide School	Range of mass media campaigns and school-based education programmes, discount schemes	✔		R	Mass media schools, health services, shops	Review Several studies reported	Observed helmet use	Increased helmet wearing rate amongst youngest children. Increased from 4.6 to 36.6% in 2 years and from 1.6 to 14% in secondary-school children 20,000 helmets sold through bulk purchase scheme	Evidence of **Reasonable** quality *Effective for some groups* Effective in younger age groups, challenge of older teenage group
Di Guiseppi et al. (1989) Bergman et al. (1990) USA	5–15 but particularly targeting elementary-school children School	Mass media campaign Community education programme School-based education programme Helmet discount scheme	✔		R	Schools, helmet manufacturers, Department of Public Health, physicians, paediatricians	Controlled trial without randomisation I = city of Seattle C = city of Portland	Observed helmet use and pre- and post-campaign helmet sales	Observed helmet wearing rates increased from 5 to 16% in the intervention sample and from 1 to 3% in the control sample (significant) Rise in helmet sales from 1500 in 1986 to 30,000 in 1989	Evidence of **Reasonable** quality *Effective for some age groups*

Table 9 (2) The road environment – bicycle helmet educational campaigns

Author, date & country	Injury target group & setting	Aims & content of intervention	Ed	Env	Leg	Healthy alliances	Study type & sample size	Outcome measures	Key results	Quality of evidence and effectiveness
Cushman, Down et al. (1991) Cushman, James et al. (1991) Canada	5–18 Primary health care	Hospital-based counselling by physicians following injury One short counselling session	✔	R		No – physicians only	Randomised controlled trial (children attending hospital after bicycling accident) I = 167 C = 172	Reported purchase/ use of helmets	Small reported increases in helmet wearing by intervention and control group (not significant)	Evidence of **Good** * quality *Inconclusive*
Morris et al. (1991) Canada	Elementary-school children School	School-based education programme helmet discount scheme (3 groups)	✔	R		School manufacturers	Randomised controlled trial (school-based) 3 school comparison 450–700 children at each school	Observed helmet use, helmet sales	No increases in helmet wearing at control and education only schools. Discounts + education only schools led to an increase from 1 to 22% pre- and post-programme (significant)	Evidence of **Reasonable** quality *Effective* The substantial subsidy of helmets was important

Table 9 (3) The road environment – bicycle helmet educational campaigns

Author, date & country	Injury target group & setting	Aims & content of intervention	Ed	Env	Leg	Healthy alliances	Study type & sample size	Outcome measures	Key results	Quality of evidence and effectiveness
Prendergast et al. (1992) USA	Elementary-school children School	School-based education programme, bicycle club discount scheme	✓		R	School PTA Retailers	Controlled trial without randomisation I = 209 C = 470	Reported behaviour Knowledge	Increased knowledge in intervention group. No increased reported helmet wearing in either group	Evidence of **Reasonable** quality *Inconclusive*
Puczynski & Marshall (1992) USA	Children 6–12 years Community-wide School	Year-long regional media campaign – Helmet distribution programme in one school & month-long education campaign Community awareness of bicycle helmets	✓		S	Local TV Newspapers Radio Hospital Schools Local athletes	Controlled trial without randomisation I = one school C = one school	Reported behaviour	After six months, in intervention school 73% of children who owned a bicycle received a helmet, reported wearing it. Compared with 23% in the comparison school	Evidence of **Reasonable/Weak** quality *Partially effective* but few details provided about baseline wearing tables
Parkin et al. (1993) Canada	5–14 years High & low income groups School	Bicycle helmet promotion programme in schools	✓		R	Schools Health professionals Retailers	Controlled trial without randomisation (n =1100)	Observed behaviour	In high income area helmet use increased from 4% to 36% in intervention group v. from 4% to 15% in control group In low income area helmet use increased from 1% to 7% in intervention group and from 3% to 13% in control group	Evidence of **Reasonable** quality *Effective for some groups*

Table 9 (4) The road environment – bicycle helmet educational campaigns

Author, date & country	Injury target group & setting	Aims & content of intervention	Ed	Env	Leg	Healthy alliances	Study type & sample size	Outcome measures	Key results	Quality of evidence and effectiveness
Schneider et al. (1993) USA	5–18 years High income group Community-wide Primary health care	Community-wide helmet promotion activities including physician counselling, discount schemes & direct to parents	✔	R		Coalition of community volunteers	Before-and-after study without control n = 595 baseline and 210 follow-up	Reported behaviour Attitudes Knowledge	Some improvements in helmet ownership Physician & telephone advice increased helmet ownership	Evidence of **weak** quality *Partially effective* Poor response rate, high attrition, biased sample

Table 10 (1) The road environment – bicycle helmet legislation

Author, date & country	Injury target group & setting	Aims & content of intervention	Ed	Env	Leg	Healthy alliances	Study type & sample size	Outcome measures	Key results	Quality of evidence and effectiveness
Dannenberg et al. (1993)	Under 16 years Middle class, rural & suburban	(First helmet law in USA) Comparison of bicycle helmet legislation (for under 16-year-olds), educational campaign & no specific campaigns in 3 counties	✓		R	✓ Schools Community group Local authorities	Controlled trial without randomisation Surveys of students in random sample of schools in 3 counties (approx. 2000 in each area)	Reported behaviour Attitudes Knowledge	Self-reported helmet use in legislation county rose from 11% to 38% after legislation, in education county from 8% to 13% and in comparison county from 7% to 11%	Evidence of **Good/ Reasonable** quality *Effective* Legislation & education more effective than education alone
Coté et al. (1992) USA	All children General population Community-wide							Observed helmet use rates	Significant increases in helmet wearing rates post-legislation in intervention community. For children increases from 4 to 47%	

Table 10 (2) The road environment – bicycle helmet legislation

Author, date & country	Injury target group & setting	Aims & content of intervention	Ed	Env	Leg	Healthy alliances	Study type & sample size	Outcome measures	Key results	Quality of evidence and effectiveness
Leicester et al. (1991)	General population	Victoria, Australia First state to introduce legislation in the world	✓	R	✓				1. Helmet wearing rates in Victoria rose from 5% in 1982/83 to 31% in 1989/90 to 75% in 1991 following law introduction	Evidence of **Good/Reasonable** quality (when all evidence taken into account *Effective*
Cameron et al. (1992)	Bicyclists in Victoria	Decade of health promotion to increase helmet use preceding legislation in July 1990					Time series of observational studies	TAC Insurance data. Hospital mortality and morbidity. Observed behaviour of bicycle use and correct helmet wearing	2. In Melbourne following legislation there was no reduction in adult cyclist exposure, moderate effect on children (10% less cyclists observed) and major effect on teenagers (decrease by 46% compared to 1990).	No control state. Some evidence of decreased exposure, particularly for teenagers, following legislation. Other major road safety initiatives (drink-driving and speeding) took place over same period and more general reductions in deaths and hospital admissions. Longer-term follow-up necessary for health outcomes
Finch et al. (1992)	Children 5–11					Wide range of agencies including schools, road organisations, police force, health care staff.	1. bicycle exposure 2. helmet wearing (sample sizes ranged from approx. 1500 to 11,000)			
Finch et al. (1993)	Teenagers 12–17	Multi-faceted campaign included Bike-Ed campaign for children 9–11	✓	R	✓				3. In Victoria there was a reduction of 48% in head injured admissions or deaths between 1989/90 and 1990/91 and 70% between 1989/90 and 1991/92.	
Vulcan et al. (1992)	Adults 18+					government organisations			(Also a reduction in non-head injuries of 23% between 1989/90 and 1990/91 and of 28% between 1990/91 and 70% between 1989/90 and 1991/92)	
Cameron et al. (1994)	Community-wide	years, bulk helmet purchase schemes, mass media publicity, efforts to improve helmet design and wide consultation Enforcement of legislation – penalties					Monitoring of insurance claims and hospital data	Observed helmet wearing		
McDermott (1995) Australia										

Table 11 (1) The road environment – child restraint and seat belt legislation

Author, date & country	Injury target group & setting	Aims & content of intervention	Ed	Env	Leg	Healthy alliances	Study type & sample size	Outcome measures	Key results	Quality of evidence and effectiveness
Decker et al. (1984) USA	Under 4 years Community-wide	Evaluation of child restraint law for under-4s in state of Tennessee		R	✓	No	Before-and-after study (series of studies)	Observed restraint use Police accident reports	Observed restraint use increased from 8% to more than 30% and deaths in children under 4 declined by 50% claimed	Evidence of **Reasonable/Weak** quality *Effective*
Guerin and MacKinnon (1985) USA	Under 3 years Community-wide	Evaluation of child restraint law for under-3s in state of California		R	✓	No	Before-and-after study with comparison area I_1 = California C_1 = non law state I_2 = children under 3 C_2 = children 4-7	Deaths and injuries recorded by police and highways departments	Injuries in target age group reduced by 8.36%. No reductions in non-target age group injuries or in comparison area	Evidence of **Reasonable** quality *Effective*
Sewell et al. (1986) USA	Under 5 years Community-wide	Evaluation of child restraint law for under-5s in State of New Mexico		R	✓	No	Before-and-after study (series of studies) I = children under 5 C = Children 5-12	Observations of restraint use and injury by police reports	Restraint use increased in target age groups from 10 to 40%; 33% reduction in fatalities and 12.6% reduction in injuries claimed	Evidence of **Reasonable** quality *Effective*
Wagenaar et al. (1986) USA	Under 4 years Community-wide	Evaluation of child restraint laws for under-4s in state of Michigan	✓	R	✓	No	Before-and-after study (series of state-wide studies) comparison groups I = children under 4 years C = children over 4 years	Observed and reported restraint use, police reports of injury	Observed restraint use for children in accidents increased from 12% to 51%; 25% decrease in injuries in target groups	Evidence of **Reasonable** quality *Effective*

Table 11 (2) The road environment – child restraint and seat belt legislation

Author, date & country	Injury target group & setting	Aims & content of intervention	Ed	Env	Leg	Healthy alliances	Study type & sample size	Outcome measures	Key results	Quality of evidence and effectiveness
Agran et al. (1987) USA	Under 4 years Community-wide	Evaluation of child restraint laws for under-4s in state of California		R	✓	No	Before-and-after study with comparison groups I = children under 4 years C = children over 4 years	Reported restraint use, hospital attendance, Coroners' reports, injury severity	Increase in reported restraint use from 26 to 50%. Decrease in injuries but no decrease in attendance at hospital	Evidence of **Reasonable** quality *Effective*
Margolis et al. (1988) USA	Under 4 years Community-wide	Evaluation of child restraint law for under-4s in Michigan		R	✓	No	Before-and-after study I = 16 Hospitals	Hospital admissions, length of hospital stay	Restraint use increased from 12 to 15% in children under 4. 36% reduction in admission for all injuries in target age group. Decline in injury severity	Evidence of **Reasonable/ Weak** quality *Effective*
Seekins et al. (1988) USA	Under 5 years Community-wide	Evaluation of child restraint laws for children in seven US states The 7 states were in different stages of the legislative process		R	✓	No	Before-and-after study – 7 state comparison	Observations of restraint use	Average increase in restraint use in target age groups from 13% to 26% (large differences between states)	Evidence of **Reasonable** quality *Partially effective* States all had different legislative requirements which makes between-state comparisons difficult

Table 11(3) The road environment – child restraint and seat belt legislation

Author, date & country	Injury target group & setting	Aims & content of intervention	Ed	Env	Leg	Healthy alliances	Study type & sample size	Outcome measures	Key results	Quality of evidence and effectiveness
Carlsson et al. (1991) Sweden	0–4 years Community-wide	1987 Restraint law for children. 6 years. Only rearward-facing seats approved	✓	R	✓	Insufficient detail	Insufficient detail (monitoring accident data) Various surveys	Mortality & morbidity data Reported behaviour Attitudes Knowledge	By 1988 40% of young children restrained in rear-facing seat and 90% restrained overall Claims differences in injury rates between rearward-facing restrained children and others	Evidence of **Weak** quality *Partially effective/ Inconclusive* (insufficient detail)
Russell et al. (1994) USA	Children under 11 years Community-wide	Intervention not directed specifically at children but study looks at effect of adult law on children's restraint use		R	✓	No	Controlled trial without randomisation C = 2699 in No Adult Law group (6 states) I = 2750 in Law group (5 states)	Reported behaviour	In I (Adult Law) 81% children under 11 years restrained compared with 74% in C (no adult law states) Adult law significant predictor of child restraint use	Evidence of **Reasonable** quality *Partially effective*

Table 12 The road environment – enforcement of legislation

Author, date & country	Injury target group & setting	Aims & content of intervention	Ed	Env	Leg	Healthy alliances	Study type & sample size	Outcome measures	Key results	Quality of evidence and effectiveness
Williams *et al.* (1987) USA	General population Community-wide	3-week programme in Elmira City, New York – special police enforcement programme to encourage seat belt use in compliance with law, printed warnings and citations + media campaigns	✓		R	Police, media	Before-and-after study with control area I= Elmira City	Process number of citations issued, observed seat belt use by front seat passengers	Seat belt use observation at baseline 49% increasing to 77% during and just after campaign and 66% two months later	Evidence of **Reasonable** quality *Effective*
Gundy (1988) Netherlands	General population Community-wide	Police enforcement and media campaign to increase seat belt use	✓		R	Police, media	Before-and-after study (5 measurement waves) with control area	Observed seat belt use and follow-up at 6 and 12 months	Improvement in seat belt use of 25% after campaign and remaining 15% above baseline at 6–12 months	Evidence of **Good/ Reasonable** quality *Effective*
Streff *et al.* (1992) USA	General population Community-wide	Public information and police enforcement campaign	✓		R	Police, researcher, media	Before-and-after campaign (several measurements 3 Michigan counties)	Observed seat belt use and number of citations issued	Observed seat belt use increased from 56.7% to 65.1% before dropping to 62.7%	Evidence of **Reasonable** quality *Partially effective*

Table 13 (1) The road environment – child restraint loan schemes

Author, date & country	Injury target group & setting	Aims & content of intervention	Ed	Env	Leg	Healthy alliances	Study type & sample size	Outcome measures	Key results	Quality of evidence and effectiveness
Reisinger et al. (1978) USA	0–1 years Primary health care	Range of interventions ranging from counselling and provision to literature to provision of free seat	✓	S		No	Before-and-after study with comparison & control groups $I_1 = 272$, $I_2 = 271$ $I_3 = 295$, $I_4 = 265$	Observed correct restraint use at discharge and 2 and 4 months	12% of those given free seat used seat correctly at discharge, this increased to 30% by 4 months. Use of seats low for all groups	Evidence of **Reasonable** quality. *Partially effective*
Christopherson et al. (1982) USA	0–1 years Primary health care	Free loan of seat and demonstration of correct use	✓	S		No	Randomised controlled trial $I = 30$ infant mother pairs	Observed correct use of restraint at discharge and 4–6 months	Correct restraint use in intervention group 67% at discharge, controls 0% correct use at discharge. No sig. differences at 4–6 months	Evidence of **Good/Reasonable** quality. *Effective* at discharge but effect not maintained
Berger et al. (1984) USA	0–1 years Low income families Primary health care	Targeted at low income families Education sessions during pre-natal, post partum & follow-up periods Free car seats provided	✓	S		Primary health care, volunteers, state agencies	Review Series of studies reported $I = 10$ hospitals	Observed correct restraint use at discharge	Increase in hospital rental schemes to cover 99% of births, Observations at discharge at 5 hospitals showed correct use increase from 15% to 70%	Evidence of **Reasonable** quality. *Effective*

Table 13 (2) The road environment – child restraint loan schemes

Author, date & country	Injury target group & setting	Aims & content of intervention	Ed	Env	Leg	Healthy alliances	Study type & sample size	Outcome measures	Key results	Quality of evidence and effectiveness
Christopherson et al. (1985) USA	0–1 years Primary health care	First ride, safe ride Hospital-based car seat loan scheme State law Group 1 education & loan scheme Group 2 – education & demonstration of correct usage	✓	✓		No	Before-and-after study. Different intervention compared I = 129	Observed correct use of restraints at discharge and 1 year	No difference between 2 groups at discharge. Correct usage rates 90% Maintained use at 80% at one year	Evidence of **Reasonable** quality *Effective* at discharge and at one year
Colletti (1986) USA	0–1 years Primary health care	Hospital-based car safety seat loan schemes across a state	✓	S		Primary health care, volunteers, state agencies	Review Series of studies reported I = 10 hospitals	Observed correct restraint use at discharge	Increase in hospital rental schemes to cover 99% of births. Observations at discharge at 5 hospitals showed correct use in increase from 15% to 70%	Evidence of **Reasonable** quality *Effective* No control groups
Geddis et al. (1986) New Zealand	0–2 years Primary health care	Car seat loan scheme to cover all newborns in city	✓			Garages, health care staff, paid co-ordinator	Before-and-after study (series of studies) No control	Yearly observations of restraint use	60–70% of parents rent infant seats from the scheme and 35–40% rent child seats. In 1981 no restraint use observed, by 1984 66% of infants restrained and 60–88% of older children	Evidence of **Weak** quality *Effective* No control groups

Table 13 (3) The road environment – child restraint loan schemes

Author, date & country	Injury target group & setting	Aims & content of intervention	Ed	Env	Leg	Healthy alliances	Study type & sample size	Outcome measures	Key results	Quality of evidence and effectiveness
Hletko et al. (1987) USA	0–1 years Primary health care	Restraint loan scheme, hospital-based programmes compared. One-to-one presentations/ counselling compared with video programme	✔			No	Comparison of 2 interventions (no controls group) I_1 = 119 I_2 = 99	Observed correct restraint use at 4 months	64.9% correct use by video programme group and 63.9% correct use by one-to-one programme group	Evidence of **Weak** quality *Inconclusive*
Jämark et al. (1988) Sweden	Inconclusive Primary health care	Free loan of seats to all parents in Swedish community for infants 0–9 months	✔	S		No I = 771	Controlled trial without randomisation C = 710	Reported behaviour	At 6 months in I 83% reported use of car restraints, 15% use of carry cots, 2% other restraints. In C after 6 months 28% reported using car restraint, 66% carry cots and 6% other restraints At 18 months 98% of I and and 95% of C were using child car restraints	Evidence of **Good*** quality *Effective* in short term (high use in both groups by 18 months)
Downing and Franklin (1989) (unpublished) UK	0–1 all children Primary health care scheme	Hospital-based child safety seat loan	✔	S		Road safety and health care staff	Before-and-after study with comparison area I_1 = Oxford I_2 = Lincoln C = Reading	Observed correct seat/ restraint use Attitudes	Decrease in lap-held infants at hospital discharge from 78 to 60% in intervention areas and increase in correct restraint use from 8 to 16%	Evidence of **Reasonable** quality *Partially effective*

Table 13 (4) The road environment – child restraint loan schemes

Author, date & country	Injury target group & setting	Aims & content of intervention	Ed	Env	Leg	Healthy alliances	Study type & sample size	Outcome measures	Key results	Quality of evidence and effectiveness
Robitaille *et al.* (1990) Canada	0–2 years (low income) Primary health care	Car seat loan scheme in low income area	✔	S		No	Comparison of intervention and comparison area I = Montreal	Observed restraint use 487 and 156 observations	Greater use of restraints observed in intervention area (41%) as compared with the control community (27%) for infants less than 6 months. No difference for older children	Evidence of **Reasonable** quality *Effective* Programme stimulated restraint use earlier but did not affect behaviour in longer term
Lindqvist (1993) Sweden	0–15 months Primary health care (0–9 months)	Hospital-based free loan scheme for infant care restraints	✔	S		No	Controlled trial without randomisation I = 937 C = 426	Self-report of injury Reported behaviour Attitudes	85% take-up rate in loan scheme; 96% of I group reported using restraint, 37% of C group used infant seats, 12% infant seats and other restraints, 50% used other types of restraints (e.g. carry cot) High rates of restraint use in both I & C after 9 months	Evidence of **Reasonable** quality *Effective* in 0–9 months

Table 14 (1) The road environment – educational campaigns for child restraint and seat belt use

Author, date & country	Injury target group & setting	Aims & content of intervention	Ed	Env	Leg	Healthy alliances	Study type & sample size	Outcome measures	Key results	Quality of evidence and effectiveness
Bass & Wilson (1964) USA	All children Primary health care	3 interventions to promote installation of seat belts in cars of patients' families Physician advice to mothers during visits (I_1) Physician's letter (I_2) Letter from safety organisation (I_3) All families exposed to ongoing TV campaign	✔		R	Safety organisations Health workers	Controlled trial without randomisation $I_1 = 221$ $I_2 = 207$ $I_3 = 530$ $C = 456$	Reported behaviour	I_1 highest % of new installation of seatbelts (43%) I_2 15% installation I_3 19% installation C 20% installation	Evidence of **Good**/ **Reasonable** quality *Partially effective* Possible bias of group more likely to visit paediatrician (I_1)
Robertson et al. (1974) USA	General population Community- wide	Media campaign to increase seat belt use. Series of TV adverts over 9 months	✔		R	No	Controlled trial without randomisation $I = 6400$ receiving cable TV $C = 7400$	Observed behaviour	Campaign had no effect on observed seat belt use. Use 12–15% in all groups before and after campaign	Evidence of **Reasonable** quality *Ineffective*

Table 14 (2) The road environment – educational campaigns for child restraint and seat belt use

Author, date & country	Injury target group & setting	Aims & content of intervention	Ed	Env	Leg	Healthy alliances	Study type & sample size	Outcome measures	Key results	Quality of evidence and effectiveness
Scherz (1976) USA	Infants Primary care	Parents attending a well-child clinic with their infants were given different educational interventions to encourage them to use infant car restraints. Control – display in clinic (I_1) – display, pamphlet (I_2) – display, pamphlet (I_3) encouraged to read pamphlet by clinic nurse (1–2 minutes) – display, pamphlet (I_4) encouraged to read pamphlet by physician (1–5 minutes) Control group	✔	R		No	Controlled trial without randomisation (not clear) $I_1 = 54$ $I_2 = 62$ $I_3 = 59$ $I_4 = 58$ $C = 52$ Series of other studies	Reported behaviour	Personal recommendations by a physician and nurse at the 4-week visit in the well-child clinic increased parent compliance by twice that of other techniques by the eighth week of life Respondents to 8-week questionnaire, contacted again at 9–12 months 96% of infants safely carried at 8 weeks, were still safely restrained at 9–12 months	Evidence of **Reasonable** / **Weak** quality *Partially effective/ inconclusive* Lack of details provided

Table 14 (3) The road environment – educational campaigns for child restraint and seat belt use

Author, date & country	Injury target group & setting	Aims & content of intervention	Ed	Env	Leg	Healthy alliances	Study type & sample size	Outcome measures	Key results	Quality of evidence and effectiveness
Miller & Pless (1977) USA	Children 1–17 years (mean 4 years) Primary care	Educational interventions in paediatrician's office to increase wearing of seat restraints 3 types of instruction (A) pamphlet alone (B) pamphlet + verbal instruction (C) pamphlet, verbal instruction + tape-slide show	✔	R		No	Randomised controlled trial IA = 82 IB = 99 IC = 215 C = 221	Reported behaviour	2 weeks after the intervention, no statistically significant changes in behaviour in any of the groups Greatest increase reported in control group	Evidence of **Good/Reasonable** quality. *Ineffective / inconclusive* Baseline behaviour was already high in intervention groups Control group behaviour lower than intervention groups – greater chance of improvement
Reisinger *et al.* (1981) USA	Infants 0–15 months Primary health care	Intervention groups received education at well child visit and targeted discussion by paediatricians with demonstration of correct use of restraints	✔	R		Primary care, well child clinics	Randomised controlled trial	Observed restraint use at 1, 2, 4 and 15 months	Correct use of restraints in the intervention group was higher at all observation points, by 23% at 1 month, 72% at 2 months, 9% at 4 months and 12% at 15 months	Evidence of **Good*** quality *Effective*
Geddis *et al.* (1982) New Zealand	Infants 0–6 months Primary health care	Educational intervention by maternity unit staff including pamphlet & film	✔	R		Primary care, maternity unit	Randomised controlled trial (sequential selection) 3 group comparison	Observed restraint use at discharge and at 6 months	Restraint use at discharge 37% and 49% among intervention groups as compared with 18% for the control group. Differences were not maintained at 6 months	Evidence of **Reasonable** quality *Partially effective* Initial improvements attributable to programme differences declined over time

Table 14 (4) The road environment – educational campaigns for child restraint and seat belt use

Author, date & country	Injury target group & setting	Aims & content of intervention	Ed	Env	Leg	Healthy alliances	Study type & sample size	Outcome measures	Key results	Quality of evidence and effectiveness
Greenberg & Coleman (1982) USA	New-born infants & their parents Hospital	Pre-natal and post partum educational programme to encourage the use of infant car restraints for first ride home from hospital. 4 groups took part: Pre-natal educational only (I_1) Pre- and post-natal (I_2) Post partum only (I_3) No education (C)	✔		R	No	Randomised controlled trial $I_1 = 27$ $I_2 = 30$ $I_3 = 11$ $C = 7$	Reported behaviour Observed behaviour	Reported and observed use of infant car restraints on trip home was highest in the group which received pre- and post-natal maternal education (but not significant) Counselling in any period associated with higher restraint use than no counselling	Evidence of **Reasonable** quality *Inconclusive* Relatively small numbers, well educated and mature group
Chang *et al.* (1985) USA	Pre-school Day care centres & nursery schools	'Buckle bear' programme In intervention group Educational programme to preschool children to increase safety seat and seat belt use and to use back seat of car. Training workshops with teachers, parent meetings, classroom lessons, films & puppets. Control group – no programme	✔		R	No	Controlled trial without randomisation (intervention & control groups carefully matched on baseline risk factors) I = 6 sites 402 children C = 7 sites 427 children	Observed behaviour Children's knowledge	Children in experimental sites increased their use of safety seats or seat belts from 21.9% to 44.3%. Control same throughout. Children also increased their knowledge and simulated practice (placing dolls in safe location in back of a toy car)	Evidence of **Good/ Reasonable** quality *Effective* Predominantly middle class, whole families targeted

Table 14 (5) The road environment – educational campaigns for child restraint and seat belt use

Author, date & country	Injury target group & setting	Aims & content of intervention	Ed	Env	Leg	Healthy alliances	Study type & sample size	Outcome measures	Key results	Quality of evidence and effectiveness
Goodson et al. (1985) USA	Infants 0–6 months Primary health care	Pre-natal child safety education targeted at parents to increase use of infant restraint seats (video + advice). Half-hour programme	✔		R	Primary care, antenatal classes	Randomised controlled trial I = 78 C = 78 (Telephone survey)	Reported restraint use at 4–6 months	(2 hospitals) intervention groups reported restraint use at 96% and 94% as compared with 78% and 60% in the control groups	Evidence of **Good*** quality *Partially effective* but reported use by control group also high
Roberts and Fanurik (1986) USA	5–11 years middle/low income areas School	School-based intervention to increase seat belt wearing for all car occupants through the application of rewards procedures. Parental involvement	✔		R	Local restaurant owner Parent volunteers 'Elephant' character Researchers School safety patrols	Before-and-after study without control I_1 = 464 I_2 = 378	Observed behaviour	In school I, compliance rates (all car occupants restrained) for seat belt wearing. 4% before intervention, 66% during intervention, 17% follow-up 1, 9% follow-up 2 School I_2 Baseline 5% during 70% follow-up 1 40% follow-up 2 20% Also increased seat belt use of drivers and other car occupants	Evidence of **Reasonable** quality *Effective* during intervention but compliance declined over time No control group

Table 14 (6) The road environment – educational campaigns for child restraint and seat belt use

Author, date & country	Injury target group & setting	Aims & content of intervention	Ed	Env	Leg	Healthy alliances	Study type & sample size	Outcome measures	Key results	Quality of evidence and effectiveness
Bowman *et al.* (1987) Australia	3–5 years School	(1) Coercion campaign aimed at parents – reminders of legislative requirements (2) Educational campaign in pre-schools with rewards for correct restraint use	✓	R		Police Pre-schools (teachers)	Controlled trial without randomisation (random school selection)	Observed seat belt use before and after intervention	Seat belt use did not improve for children in the parent coercion or control groups. Significant improvements in seat belt use were reported by the education group (use increased from 61 to 75%)	Evidence of **Reasonable** quality *Effective*
Macknin *et al.* (1987) USA	Children and teenagers 5–19 attending well child appointments Primary health care	Paediatricians promoted seat belt use at private well child appointment + follow-up at 12 months	✓	R		No	Randomised controlled study (sequential group selection) I = 242 C = 77	Observed seat belt use at 12-month telephone follow-up	38% increase in seat belt use after intervention for those not belted before. (5% increase by controls) No differences at 12-month follow-up between the groups	Evidence of **Good*** quality *Effective* initially but no long-term effect
Sowers *et al.* (1987) USA	Children 4–7 years School	Small-scale study, educational programme, school-based with rewards and prizes for seat belt use by children Group 1 programme of 26 days Group 2 programme of 14 days	✓	R		No	2 group comparison before and after (16 children observed not wearing belts) I₁=8 I₂=8	Observed seat belt use	At baseline no children were wearing seat belts. After the programme seat belt use increased to 96% for Group 1 and 81% for Group 2. At 2 months 86% of Group 1 used seat belts and 75% of Group 2	Evidence of **Reasonable/ Weak** quality *Effective* but numbers in 2 groups are very small

Table 14 (7) The road environment – educational campaigns for child restraint and seat belt use

Author, date & country	Injury target group & setting	Aims & content of intervention	Ed	Env	Leg	Healthy alliances	Study type & sample size	Outcome measures	Key results	Quality of evidence and effectiveness
Thyer *et al.* (1987) USA	General population (front seat passenger) Community-wide	Small-scale study looking at the effects of a dashboard sticker on seat belt use by front seat passengers	✔	R		No	Before-and-after study (ABAB time series design) I = 24	Observed seat belt use	Seat belt use increased from 34–41% at baselines to 70–78% with stickers present	Evidence of **Reasonable** quality *Effective* General population but relatively simple intervention producing positive results
Roberts *et al.* (1988) USA	Elementary school children) 5–14 years Schools	Community-wide programme through schools, educational campaign with rewards for children	✔	R		Schools PTAs Businesses Local authorities	Before-and-after study, no control (observations at randomly selected schools) I = 25 schools	Observed seat belt use at 3 schools	Rewards increased seat belt use during the campaign from 18.1% at baseline to 62.4% during and 49% after the campaign and the withdrawal of rewards	Evidence of **Reasonable** quality *Effective*
Morrow (1989) USA	Children 4–8 years & their parents School	'May is Buckle-up Month' programme. School-based curricular intervention for young children to improve seat belt use in cars in one-month intervention	✔	R		No	Before-and-after study I = 422 children Pre-intervention 125 children 132 drivers observed After intervention 147 children 150 adults observed At one-month follow-up 107 children 107 adults	Observed behaviour by children and parents	Seat belt use in children increased from 46% to 66% and stayed at 63% at 1 month Parent use improved from 47% to 61% and 62% at 1-month follow-up	Evidence of **Reasonable/ Weak** quality *Effective* but only one school and no control group

Table 14 (8) The road environment – educational campaigns for child restraint and seat belt use

Author, date & country	Injury target group & setting	Aims & content of intervention	Ed	Env	Leg	Healthy alliances	Study type & sample size	Outcome measures	Key results	Quality of evidence and effectiveness
Neuwelt et al. (1989) USA	15–19 Secondary school teenagers School	Educational intervention to encourage seat belt use school-based – films, experts, literature	✔	R		Schools Primary care	Controlled trial without randomisation (matched pre- and post-surveys) I= 4 schools C=3 schools	Observed seat belt use Knowledge Attitudes	Increased knowledge following intervention but no change in observed seat belt use on exit from school parking lots	Evidence of quality *Inconclusive*
Stuy et al. (1993) USA	2–6 years Low socio-economic group Primary health care	Programme in child care centres to encourage routine correct use of child restraints. Involving centre-staff training letter to parents, age-appropriate classroom activities for children	✔	R		✔ Child care staff University Parents	Randomised controlled trial Unit of randomisation = centre I=71 families 94 children C=120 families 139 children	Observed behaviour Knowledge	Increase in restraint use at intervention centre from 54% to 75% Control centre maintained low use of restraints (range 20–30%)	Evidence of **Reasonable** quality *Partially effective* Reservations about differences of control and intervention groups Results difficult to interpret

Table 15 The home environment – prevention of other specific home accidents

Author, date & country	Injury target group & setting	Aims & content of intervention	Ed	Env	Leg	Healthy alliances	Study type & sample size	Outcome measures	Key results	Quality of evidence and effectiveness
Kravitz (1973) USA	0–1 years Primary health care	Parent counselling by paediatrician on dangers of falls in infancy	✔			No	Controlled trial without randomisation I=320 C=366	Accident reports	Significant differences between intervention group having less injuries (17.2% control group v. 10.3% intervention)	Evidence of **Reasonable** quality *Effective*
Spiegel *et al.* (1977) USA	All children Community-wide	(Targeted at window falls) (1) injury surveillance (2) Counselling by nurses (3) Mass media campaign (4) Home visits, hazard identification (5) Provision of free window guards	✔	S	✔	Police, primary health care, community groups	Before-and-after study without control	Deaths and injuries (police and hospital reports)	35% decrease in mortality due to falls City-wide decrease in falls of 31% 16,000 free guards provided to 4200 families	Evidence of **Reasonable/ Weak** quality *Effective*
Kraus (1985) USA	All children Community-wide	Evaluation of product redesign to prevent suffocation and strangulation by refrigerator entrapment, crib deaths and suffocation by plastic bags	✔	✔		Manufacturers, legislature	Before-and-after study (time series)	Deaths (statistics available from 1960 to 1981)	Significant decline in refrigerator entrapment deaths and plastic bag suffocations. Declining numbers of crib suffocations	Evidence of **Reasonable** quality *Effective* Preventive measures introduced may have been responsible for the reduction in suffocation and strangulation deaths

Table 16 (1) The home environment – prevention of general home accidents

Author, date & country	Injury target group & setting	Aims & content of intervention	Ed	Env	Leg	Healthy alliances	Study type & sample size	Outcome measures	Key results	Quality of evidence and effectiveness
Schlesinger et al. (1966) USA	Under 7 Community-wide	Health education through network of neighbourhood groups Literature provided	✔			Community-wide/ primary health care	Controlled trial without randomisation I=4041 C=4063	All medically attended injuries	No differences between intervention and control groups in terms of medically attended injury rates	Evidence of **Reasonable** quality *Inconclusive/ ineffective*
Dershewitz et al. (1977) USA	Under 5 Primary health care	20-minute personalised counselling, literature on prevention of injuries. Outlet covers and door catches provided free	✔	S		No	Randomised controlled trial I=100 C=100	Observed behaviour, attitudes and knowledge	No difference between intervention and control groups in terms of observed hazards. Some evidence of safety proofing in intervention group (70% made at least one change)	Evidence of **Good*** quality *Inconclusive/ partially effective*
Dershewitz (1979) USA	Under 5 Primary health care	Intervention group received education, both control and intervention groups received free safety devices – socket covers and cupboard catches and instructions	✔	S		No	Randomised controlled trial I=101 C=104	Observed behaviour	Significant increase in the use of outlet covers in both groups but not cupboard catches which took more effort to install	Evidence of **Good*** quality *Partially effective*
Colver et al. (1982) UK	Under 5 Low socio-economic area Home Community-wide	Locally designed health education initiative and mass media campaign Home visits where specific advice given on hazard reduction	✔	R		No	Randomised controlled trial I=43 families C=37 families	Observed behaviour	60% of the intervention group made some physical change to make their homes safe as compared with 9% of the control group	Evidence of **Good*** quality *Effective*

Table 16 (2) The home environment – prevention of general home accidents

Author, date & country	Injury target group & setting	Aims & content of intervention	Ed	Env	Leg	Healthy alliances	Study type & sample size	Outcome measures	Key results	Quality of evidence and effectiveness
Minchom et al. (1984) UK	All children Community-wide	(General home accidents) Health education campaign, talks, literature and health visitor visits to 'at risk' households	✔			Community groups, schools, primary health care	Controlled trial without randomisation I = community in Cardiff C = rest of city	Injuries (A & E attendances)	No significant differences in accident from the pre- to post-intervention and control areas	Evidence of **Reasonable** quality *Ineffective*
Gallagher et al. (1985) USA	Under 6 Home Community-wide	(Part of SCIPP programme) Home visits to assess hazards (1) enforcement of sanitary code (2) safety inspection and counselling (3) distribution of safety devices	✔	S		Schools, fire services, local officials, hospital	Before-and-after study I = 285 households	Observed behaviour	Tap water temperatures were 11% cooler at follow-up. Some reduction of other hazards. No improvements in some areas	Evidence of **Reasonable/ Weak** quality *Partially effective*
Barone et al. (1986) USA	Under 5 Families with child abuse blame Home	Home visits by family counsellors to identify hazards. Intensive training programme. Cupboard locks provided	✔	S		No	Case study 3 families No controls	Observed behaviour	Consistent reduction in observed hazards – safety latches fitted Improvements maintained over time	Evidence of **Weak** quality *Partially effective*

Table 16 (3) The home environment – prevention of general home accidents

Author, date & country	Injury target group & setting	Aims & content of intervention	Ed	Env	Leg	Healthy alliances	Study type & sample size	Outcome measures	Key results	Quality of evidence and effectiveness
Kelly et al. (1987) USA	0–1 (well child attendances) Primary health care	15-minute individualised counselling in child safety at 3 well child visits	✓	R		No	Randomised controlled trial I= 85 C= 86	Reported accidents, observed and reported behaviour Knowledge	No change in accidents reported. Improvement in certain safety practices and some improvement in knowledge in intervention group	Evidence of Good/ **Reasonable** quality *Partially effective*
Baudier et al. (1988) France	Pre-school & kindergarten children Home	Education programme or pre-school & kindergarten children using kit prepared by French committee for health education. Information provided for parents	✓			No	Controlled trial without randomisation I= 20 schools C= 20 schools	Knowledge Attitudes Reported behaviour (Children, parents & teachers)	Changes in parental (reported) behaviour about storage of medicines and household cleaning products. Teachers positive about the programme.	Evidence of **Reasonable** quality *Partially effective* but relatively few details provided
DTI (1989) UK	General population	(Hazard dome) Evaluation of a DTI audio-visual exhibition designed to increase awareness of home accidents	✓			No	Before-and-after study	Knowledge awareness	Reinforced the belief that the home is a dangerous place for young children. Enhanced awareness of specific dangers	Evidence of **Weak** quality *Partially effective*

Table 16 (4) The home environment – prevention of general home accidents

Author, date & country	Injury target group & setting	Aims & content of intervention	Ed	Env	Leg	Healthy alliances	Study type & sample size	Outcome measures	Key results	Quality of evidence and effectiveness
Sullivan *et al.* (1990) USA	Under 6 Targeted at burn victims Home	Home visits to identify hazards plus specific recommendations. Some devices provided bath thermometers, poison stickers	✔	S		Burn centre, health visitors	Before-and-after study (targeted at burn victims) I=21	Observed behaviour	Parents complied with 43.5% of the total recommendations plus positive effects on home hazards	Evidence of **Weak** quality *Partially effective*
DTI (1992b) UK	General population	(Giant trailer) Evaluation of a DTI audio-visual exhibiton designed to increase awareness of home accidents	✔			No	Controlled trial without randomisation	Knowledge/ awareness	Short-term impact on awareness of hazards	Evidence of **Reasonable** quality *Partially effective* *Partially effective*
Paul *et al.* (1994) Australia	10 months – 2 years Home	Safe Place Project Intervention by trained volunteers involving home visits and aiming to reduce home safety hazards & increase knowledge	✔	R		Researchers Volunteers Safety shows Hospital	Randomised controlled trial I= 94 families C= 104 Post-test I= 48 C=58	Observation of hazards Knowledge	Decrease in hazards pre- and post-intervention in intervention group At post-test no significant differences for hazards cores in I and C groups. Increase in knowledge in intervention group	Evidence of **Reasonable** quality *Unclear/ inconclusive* Sample attrition large No control pre-tests

Table 16 (5)   The home environment – prevention of general home accidents

Author, date & country	Injury target group & setting	Aims & content of intervention	Ed	Env	Leg	Healthy alliances	Study type & sample size	Outcome measures	Key results	Quality of evidence and effectiveness
Olds *et al.* (1994) USA	Pre-school children of teenaged or poor women	Nurse home visitations during pregnancy and first two years of life I Four groups (1) when children aged 1–2 screened for sensory & developmental problems & referred (2) free transport provided pre-natal & well child care at local clinics + screening in (1) (3) in addition to (1) & (2) families provided with nurse home visitor – average 9 visits (4) in addition to (1),(2) &(3) nurse continued to visit until child was 2	✓			No	Randomised controlled trial C_1 } $= 129$ C_2 $I_3 = 73$ $I_4 = 80$ Numbers used in analysis relating to home and car safety	Observed hazards Reported behaviour	At 34 months and 46 months in home assessment, homes of nurse visited families (groups 3 & 4) had fewer hazards than homes where there had been no nurse visits. No programme influences on extent to which mothers reported poisonous substances were kept out of reach of children or reported use of child safety restraints in cars	Evidence of **Reasonable** quality Injury outcomes part of larger study – not very much detail provided. *Partially effective*

Table 17 (1) The home environment – prevention of burns and scalds

Author, date & country	Injury target group & setting	Aims & content of intervention	Ed	Env	Leg	Healthy alliances	Study type & sample size	Outcome measures	Key results	Quality of evidence and effectiveness
Sørensen (1976) Denmark	General population Community-wide	Identification of 3 specific burn injuries led to 3 interventions (1) launderette washers (2) vacuum cleaners (3) coffee filters Lobbying manufacturers, safer design, new regulations	✔	✔	✔	Hospitals State Manufacturers	Before-and-after study without control	Observed behaviour Mortality and morbidity data	(1) Eradication of burn injuries associated with front-loading launderette washers (2) Vacuum cleaner and coffee filter injuries reduced	Evidence of **Reasonable** quality *Effective* Good example of the effects of redesign of consumer products on injury rates
Linares & Linares (1979) USA	8–13 years School	Single multimedia lecture on burn injury prevention – feedback on test results to reinforce learning	✔			No	Before-and-after study without control I = 67	Knowledge	Increase in knowledge for all questions and age groups	Evidence of **Reasonable**/ **Weak** quality *Effective* but no evidence that knowledge affects behaviour

Table 17 (2) The home environment – prevention of burns and scalds

Author, date & country	Injury target group & setting	Aims & content of intervention	Ed	Env	Leg	Healthy alliances	Study type & sample size	Outcome measures	Key results	Quality of evidence and effectiveness
McLoughlin et al. (1979)	General population (components aimed at children)	Project Burn Prevention Large community-wide public education programme	✓			Schools Police Consumer organisations Community leaders Medical institutions	Controlled trial without randomisation (community-wide by area)	Mortality & morbidity data (death records and hospital records) Knowledge Reported behaviour	Knowledge gains demonstrated from schools programme but no reduction in burn injuries. Community comparison may have led to a short-term reduction in injuries. There was an increase in the rate of burn injuries for the media campaign area, explained possibly by random variation in burn incidence	Evidence of **Reasonable** quality *Partially effective/ inconclusive*
McLoughlin et al. (1982)	Community-wide	to reduce burn injuries. Mass media, school and community programme								
MacKay & Rothman (1982) USA	School	One community – school-based programme Second community – community-wide campaign								
Miller et al. (1982) USA	All children (well child visits) Primary health care	Paediatrician counselling at well child sessions to reduce burn injuries. Smoke detectors available at cost price	✓	R		No	Randomised controlled trial I=120 C=120	Observed behaviour	Significant increase in detectors installed in intervention households – 25/55 installed detectors no control group changes	Evidence of **Good*** quality *Effective*

Table 17 (3) The home environment – prevention of burns and scalds

Author, date & country	Injury target group & setting	Aims & content of intervention	Ed	Env	Leg	Healthy alliances	Study type & sample size	Outcome measures	Key results	Quality of evidence and effectiveness
Thomas *et al.* (1984) USA	Pre-school (well baby clinic) Primary health care	Burns and scalds targeted (1) education session (2) discount coupons for smoke detectors at well child sessions	✓	R		No	Randomised controlled trial I = 29 C = 29	Observed behaviour	65% of intervention group had safe hot water temperatures at follow-up visit. None of control group had safe temperatures. No difference in operational smoke detectors across groups	Evidence of **Good/Reasonable** quality *Partially effective*
Eckelt *et al.* (1985) USA	Elementary school children School	Brief one-hour burn prevention programme in schools	✓			Burns unit staff Fire chief Social worker	Before-and-after study without control I = 299	Knowledge	Significant improvements in mean post-test scores (from 66.3% to 79.9%)	Evidence of **Reasonable/ Weak** quality *Effective* applicable in both public and private schools
McLoughlin *et al.* (1985) USA	General population Community-wide	Evaluation of smoke detector legislation 5 years after its introduction	✓	R		Fire department Primary health care	Controlled trial without randomisation I = 500 C = 400	(Deaths) Observed behaviour	Similar rates of detectors in both communities. Reductions in deaths greater in intervention community	Evidence of **Good/Reasonable** quality *Partially effective/ inconclusive*
Elberg *et al.* (1987) Denmark	General population (component aimed at under 5 years) Community-wide	Ongoing national educational campaign over 17-year period to reduce incidence of burns and scalds	✓	✓	✓	Mass media Government Industry (few details)	Time series? (monitors burns over 17-year period)	Mortality & morbidity data	Overall downward trend in burn hospitalisations. This was particularly marked in under-5 group	Evidence of **Weak** quality *Possibly effective in some groups/ inconclusive* No evidence that outcomes are attributable to the intervention.(little detail provided)

Table 17 (4) The home environment – prevention of burns and scalds

Author, date & country	Injury target group & setting	Aims & content of intervention	Ed	Env	Leg	Healthy alliances	Study type & sample size	Outcome measures	Key results	Quality of evidence and effectiveness
Varas et al. (1988) USA	Elementary school age / School	Brief one-hour burn prevention programme in schools with specific messages	✓			Fire service Schools nurse	Before-and-after study without control I= 69 schools	Knowledge	At pre-test only 1% of children could answer all questions correctly, at post-test this had risen to 61%	Evidence of **Reasonable** quality *Effective* No controls
Katcher et al. (1989) USA	All children – particularly under 3 years / Primary health care	Intervention involving health care counselling and literature on safe domestic hot water temperature. I received free thermometer to check water temperatures. Home visits to check temperatures in a sample	✓	R		No	Randomised controlled trial I=315 C=347	Observed behaviour Reported behaviour Knowledge	12% of subjects reported lowering water temperature but no significant difference between I and C. No differences between groups in terms of knowledge. 73% gained knowledge after the intervention	Evidence of **Good*** quality *Partially effective*
Webne et al. (1989) USA	Under 9	Targeted at families with high temperatures – thermometers provided	✓	S		No	Before-and-after study I= 12 families	Observed behaviour	No statistically significant decrease in water temperature	Evidence of **Weak** quality *Inconclusive*

Table 17 (5) The home environment – prevention of burns and scalds

Author, date & country	Injury target group & setting	Aims & content of intervention	Ed	Env	Leg	Healthy alliances	Study type & sample size	Outcome measures	Key results	Quality of evidence and effectiveness
Erdmann et al. (1991) USA	All children Community-wide	10-year evaluation of state law requiring new water heaters to be preset at 49°C. Random survey to check whether water heaters had been adjusted				Water heater manufacturers	Before-and-after study and random survey of water temperatures	Burn injuries (hospital admission) Observed behaviour	56% reduction in admissions for burns. Significant reduction in water temperatures	Evidence of **Reasonable** quality *Effective*
Hammond & Varas (1990) USA	General population (high-risk neighbour-hoods) Community-wide	Buy one – give one free Community smoke detector give-away programme. Free smoke detector given to low income families. Smoke detectors installed & checked	✔	S		Community-wide Fire department Local organisations Chamber of Commerce Burn centre	Before-and-after study without control	Observed behaviour	6000 smoke detectors sold by community organisations 6000 fitted free in low income households. Impact on morbidity/ mortality unclear	Evidence of **Reasonable/ Weak** quality *Effective* (little detail provided)
Laing & Bryant (1991) New Zealand	All children Community-wide	Safety of Children's Nightwear Act (1987) Legislative intervention to reduce children's burn injuries from nightwear	✔	✔	No		Before-and-after study without control	Hospital admissions	A very downward trend for nightwear burn incidence. (Other possible explanations for injury reductions)	Evidence of **Weak** quality *Effective* outcomes may not be wholly attributable to interventions

Table 17 (6) The home environment – prevention of burns and scalds

Author, date & country	Injury target group & setting	Aims & content of intervention	Ed	Env	Leg	Healthy alliances	Study type & sample size	Outcome measures	Key results	Quality of evidence and effectiveness
Grant *et al.* (1992) USA	8–9 years School	Learn Not to Burn Programme Burn prevention programme through state schools. Materials produced by fire service 22 key behaviours targeted	✓			Schools Fire service Insurance companies	Randomised controlled trial (schools unit of randomisation) I=20 school districts C=10 school districts	Knowledge	No significant differences between school districts. High baseline score	Evidence of **Good/ Reasonable** quality *Ineffective*
Thompson *et al.* (1992) USA	12–14 years School	School-based burn prevention programme aimed at teenagers as potential baby sitters. Brief, one-off slide presentation	✓			No	Before-and-after study without control. I=119	Knowledge	No significant difference at pre- and post-test. Little new information learned by students	Evidence of **Weak** quality *Ineffective* An interesting target group. Weak evaluation of a short intervention

Table 17 (7) The home environment – prevention of burns and scalds

Author, date & country	Injury target group & setting	Aims & content of intervention	Ed	Env	Leg	Healthy alliances	Study type & sample size	Outcome measures	Key results	Quality of evidence and effectiveness
Fallat & Rengers (1993) USA	Under 5 years High-risk area Community-wide	National Safe Kids campaign Pilot project by local coalition to provide education & anti-scald devices to prevent burns in pre-school children Intervention by health care workers	✔	S		Safe kids coalition Hospitals Housing authorities	Before-and-after study without control I₁ = 60 I₂=20	Hospital admissions Observed behaviour Knowledge	Survey knowledge increased after intervention and some knowledge retention after 18 months Poor performance of scald-burn devices At 9 months 17/20 removed due to build-up of sediment Claimed small reductions in scald burns	Evidence of **Reasonable/Weak** quality *Partially effective/ inconclusive* No evidence that injury outcomes attributable to intervention
Waller *et al.* (1993) New Zealand	Pre-school targeted at children under 3 Community-wide	'Hot water burns like Fire' programme National mass media campaign and local pilot projects including community lobbying for building code legislation for safe water temperatures. Home education and water temperature measured by health staff in some areas	✔	S	✔	Yes Mass media Community groups Health care staff Insurance companies	Randomised controlled trial I = 54 C = 56	Observed behaviour Attitudes and Knowledge	There was a significant decrease in hot water temperatures in both groups after the campaigns, nevertheless temperatures remained unsafe in the majority of households	Evidence of **Good/ Reasonable** quality *Partially effective* Water heating systems in many homes were not amenable to the intervention

Table 17 (8) The home environment – prevention of burns and scalds

Author, date & country	Injury target group & setting	Aims & content of intervention	Ed	Env	Leg	Healthy alliances	Study type & sample size	Outcome measures	Key results	Quality of evidence and effectiveness
Lewis *et al.* (1994) USA	8–9 years School	Learn Not to Burn Programme Burn prevention programme through schools. Brief presentation to large groups.	✓			No	Before-and-after study without controls I = 17 schools 700 children	Knowledge	Some reported improvement in scores	Evidence of **Weak** quality *Inconclusive*

Table 18 (1) The home environment – prevention of poisoning

Author, date & country	Injury target group & setting	Aims & content of intervention	Ed	Env	Leg	Healthy alliances	Study type & sample size	Outcome measures	Key results	Quality of evidence and effectiveness
Maisel & Langdoc (1967) USA	Under 5 years Community-wide	Community-wide Multi-faceted programme to reduce poisoning by parent & child education	✔			Community-wide	Before-and-after study without control. Before 604 After 1129 questionnaires	Knowledge Reported behaviour Hospital admissions	Claim reductions of 23–29%in poison admissions. Results inconclusive for knowledge and reported behaviour	Evidence of **Weak** quality *Unclear/ inconclusive* Detail on reach and process. No control, high levels of inappropriate behaviour
Dershewitz et al. (1983) USA	9-month-old Primary health care	Pediatrician counselling at routine well child visits on appropriate use of ipecac & management of poisonings (ipecac supplied)	✔	S		No	Before-and-after study without control I=78	Knowledge	Significant increase in knowledge related to caustic ingestion. Overall 51% improved, 19% had worse score post-intervention	Evidence of **Weak** quality *Partially effective* but worse scores in some. No control group
Dershewitz & Paichel (1984) USA	9–11 month infants Lower socio-economic Primary health care	Nurse practitioner counselling at routine well child visits on appropriate use of ipecac & management of poisonings (ipecac supplied)	✔	S		No	Before-and-after study without control I=69	Knowledge	56% mothers improved scores & 22% had worse scores. Knowledge gain less than higher social group in Dershewitz (1983). Intervention potentially harmful	Evidence of **Weak** quality *Inconclusive/ potentially harmful* Insufficient detail on intervention

Table 18 (2) The home environment – prevention of poisoning

Author, date & country	Injury target group & setting	Aims & content of intervention	Ed	Env	Leg	Healthy alliances	Study type & sample size	Outcome measures	Key results	Quality of evidence and effectiveness
Sibert et al. (1985) UK	Under 5 years Community-wide	Voluntary agreement by pharmaceutical industry 1981 – packaging of solid dose medications in CRCs or blister packs		✓	✓	Government Pharmaceutical industry	Before-and-after study without control	Hospital admissions	No significant fall in hospital admissions over 5-year study period. Steady increase in poisoning with liquid preparations	Evidence of **Reasonable** quality *Partially effective* many substances not dispensed in CRCs
Woolf et al. (1987) USA	Under 5 years Primary health care	Emergency room counselling by medical staff on poison management (supplied ipecac)	✓	S		No	Randomised controlled trial I = 119 C_1 = 83 C_2 = 60 (59% completed follow-up)	Knowledge Reported behaviour	Storage of ipecac increased from 37% to 68% in I From 29% to 47% in C1 In C_2 36% at follow-up. Significant difference in intervention group	Evidence of **Reasonable** quality *Partially effective* but little knowledge of how to use ipecac. Differences at baseline between I and C1
Woolf (1992) USA	Under 5 years (families without ipecac) Home	Mailed package intervention by poison centre staff for families seeking advice after poisoning incidents. Cabinet lock provided	✓	S		No	Randomised controlled trial I = 169 150 F/U C = 167 151 F/U	Self-report of injury Reported behaviour	Intervention group more likely to report presence of telephone sticker and use of storage lock. No differences in availability of ipecac other reported poison and behaviour. No difference in poisoning recurrence but short follow-up period. Money-off coupons did not work	Evidence of **Reasonable** quality *Partially effective* (sample of poison centre callers predominately white and well educated)

Table 18 (3) The home environment – prevention of poisoning

Author, date & country	Injury target group & setting	Aims & content of intervention	Ed	Env	Leg	Healthy alliances	Study type & sample size	Outcome measures	Key results	Quality of evidence and effectiveness
Schnell (1993) USA	80% 1–3 years (families calling poison centre) High education level Home	Mailed package intervention from poison centre. Ipecac supplied	✔	S		No	Before-and-after study without control I = 100 90 F/U	Knowledge Reported behaviour	At enrolment 47% had ipecac and 51% knew purpose. At follow-up 94% had ipecac and 92 % knew purpose	Evidence of **Weak** quality *Effective* but target group already motivated No control group
Krug *et al.* (1994) South Africa	Under 5 Primary health care	Free distribution by health workers of CRCs for paraffin storage to parents and awareness raising	✔	S		Health workers Research team Shell SA	Controlled trial without randomisation. 20,000 CRCs distributed	Hospital clinic data for mortality & morbidity. Observed & reported behaviour Attitudes Knowledge	Distribution of CRCs in study area reduced incidence of paraffin ingestion by 47% (no change in control area)	Evidence of **Good*** quality *Effective* but problem of intermediate containers needs to be addressed Cost of containers high

Table 19 The leisure environment – prevention of sports and leisure injuries

Author, date & country	Injury target group & setting	Aims & content of intervention	Ed	Env	Leg	Healthy alliances	Study type & sample size	Outcome measures	Key results	Quality of evidence and effectiveness
Morton & Burton (1975) New Zealand	High school School	School-based programme. Rugby players provided with mouth guards in attempt to reduce dental injury	✔	S		Schools Dentists	Before-and-after study without control. I = 272 (221 F/U)	Morbidity data Self-report of injury Reported behaviour	61% reported wearing mouth guards regularly and 30% occasionally. 14% suffered dental injury during season. The difference between mouth guard wearers and non-wearers was significant	Evidence of **Reasonable** quality *Effective* (no controls) Some evidence that device needed modification

Table 20 General mass media campaigns

Author, date & country	Injury target group & setting	Aims & content of intervention	Ed	Env	Leg	Healthy alliances	Study type & sample size	Outcome measures	Key results	Quality of evidence and effectiveness
Williams & Sibert (1983) UK	Under 15 years Community-wide	1st BBC TV series *Play it Safe*	✔			Mass media	Before-and-after study	Hospital admissions (for burns and scalds and fractured femurs)	No significant difference before and after TV series	Evidence of **Reasonable**/ **Weak** quality *Ineffective/ inconclusive*
Naidoo (1984) UK	Under 7 years Community-wide	1st BBC TV series *Play it Safe* and local child injury prevention group	✔			Mass media, health visitors	Before-and-after study	Accident and emergency attendance	No significant difference before and after TV series	Evidence of **Weak** quality *Ineffective/ inconclusive*
Banbury (1992) UK	All children Community-wide	2nd BBC TV series *Play it Safe* Mass media campaign with support literature	✔			Mass media	Before-and-after study Before 1000 questioned After 3000 questioned	Penetration of broadcasts Knowledge Reported behaviour	Audience figures 8.8–9.6 million. 240,000 booklets distributed Increased reported safer behaviour, e.g. installing smoke detector increased from 38% to 43%	**Reasonable**/ **Weak** quality *Effective*

Table 21 (1) Community-based studies

Author, date & country	Injury target group & setting	Aims & content of intervention	Ed	Env	Leg	Healthy alliances	Study type & sample size	Outcome measures	Key results	Quality of evidence and effectiveness
Tellnes (1985) Norway	General population Community-wide	Community-based Health education based on local information delivered by GPs, child health and school clinics	✔			General practice Mass media Unions School Fishermen Health services	Before-and-after study I = Vaery & Rost (pop 1068)	Consultations with physician Hospital admissions	No reduction in first year plus 29% reduction claimed in second year	Evidence of **Weak** quality *Inconclusive* No controls Few details provided
Robertson (1986) USA	General population Community-wide	Community-based programme alongside national campaign. Focused on first-aid training, smoke detectors, child restraints in cars	✔	✔		Environmental health Clinical staff Community representatives	Before-and-after study without control Injury rates calculated	Hospital admissions	Claimed reductions in hospital admissions for falls, motor vehicle injuries and assaults	Evidence of **Weak** quality *Inconclusive* No controls No evidence that outcomes attributable to intervention
Schelp (1987)	General population Community-wide	Health promotion based on local community diagnosis Home and work environment targeted Range of intervention	✔	R		Child health care and welfare Multi-agency	Controlled trial without randomisation I = Falköping C = Linköping	Accident and emergency admissions, deaths	Reduction of 27% in home accidents and 28% in occupational accidents	Evidence of **Reasonable** quality *Effective*
Guyer et al. (1989) USA	Under 5 Community-wide	Health promotion campaigns based on 5 interventions: prevention of burns, poisonings, falls, suffocations and passenger RTSs	✔	R		Multi-agency Mass media Schools	Controlled trial without randomisation I = 9 communities C = 5 communities	Accident and emergency attendance Reported behaviour Knowledge	Reduction in motor vehicle occupant injuries but not in other injury areas 42% of households in I communities exposed to at least one intervention	Evidence of **Good*** quality *Effective* for some elements of campaign

Table 21 (2) Community-based studies

Author, date & country	Injury target group & setting	Aims & content of intervention	Ed	Env	Leg	Healthy alliances	Study type & sample size	Outcome measures	Key results	Quality of evidence and effectiveness
Sahlin & Lereim (1990) Norway	Under 7 years Community-wide	Health promotion based on local community diagnosis. Two-year programme. Nurse counselling targeted advice	✓			Child health care	Before-and-after study I= Trondheim	Hospital admissions	Reduction in accidents 3.4% fewer days of hospitalisation after intervention	Evidence of **Weak** quality *Inconclusive* No controls Few details provided
Bass et al. (1991) Bass et al. (1985) USA	Under 5 years Community-wide	Paediatric counselling programme and SCIPP interventions (burns, falls, poisoning, car occupant injuries)	✓			Paediatricians	Before-and-after controlled study of communities I = 4 communities C= suburban community	Accident and emergency attendance	Claimed 15.3% decrease in injury	Evidence of **Reasonable** quality *Partially effective* May have been cross-contamination with this and target SCIPP study
Jeffs et al. (1993) Australia	Under 14 years Community-wide	Community approach based on Falköping model focused on backyard clean-ups & bicycle campaigns. Activities included: rubbish collection and trial of ECIPP (see Walker et al., 1991). Bicycle helmet legislation introduced in state during campaign	✓	✓	✓	Intersectoral task force including police, traffic, community & health organisations. 26 organisations	Before-and-after study without control Hospital records monitored	Hospital admission and attendance Knowledge	Number of injuries relating to backyard junk fell from 14% of presentations to 7%. Bicycle-related injuries fell from 11% of child attendances in 1987 to 7% in 1991	Evidence of **Reasonable/ Weak** quality *Inconclusive* No control No evidence that outcomes attributable to campaign

Table 21 (3) Community-based studies

Author, date & country	Injury target group & setting	Aims & content of intervention	Ed	Env	Leg	Healthy alliances	Study type & sample size	Outcome measures	Key results	Quality of evidence and effectiveness
Schwarz et al. (1993) USA	General population Focus on urban African American Community-wide	Safe Block Project Intervention by community workers involving home inspections and educational programme. Package of home safety devices supplied Emphasis on falls, fires, scalds, poisonings and violence prevention	✔	✔		Dept of Public Health Safety Inspectors Community volunteers	Controlled trial without randomisation I = 3004 C = 1472	Observation of hazards Knowledge	Block representatives recruited for 88% of blocks. Intervention homes significantly more likely to have ipecac and smoke detectors. No consistent differences for home hazards requiring major efforts. Distinct difference between intervention and control homes in safety knowledge	Evidence of **Good/ Reasonable** quality *Partially effective* No baseline data on control groups
Davidson et al. (1994) USA	5–16 years Disadvantaged community	Safe Kids/Healthy Neighborhoods Injury Prevention Programme Community-wide interventions targeting RTAs, outdoor falls and violence. Involved playground renovation, education and supervised activities	✔			26 organisations city agencies voluntary organisations, citizens' groups	Controlled trial without randomisation Community-wide target I = Central Harlem C = Washington Heights	Mortality and morbidity data	Significant reductions in injuries in intervention and control areas. In intervention area claimed 44% reduction in targeted injuries. In intervention areas decline was specific to targeted injuries	Evidence of **Reasonable** quality *Partially effective/ inconclusive* Characteristics of I and C areas different and evidence of injury reduction in both areas
Kuhn et al. (1994) USA	Community-wide									

Table 21 (4) Community-based studies

Author, date & country	Injury target group & setting	Aims & content of intervention	Ed	Env	Leg	Healthy alliances	Study type & sample size	Outcome measures	Key results	Quality of evidence and effectiveness
Ozanne-Smith et al. (1994) Australia	All ages Community-wide	Shire of Bulla Safe Living Program All age, all injury type community programme based on Falköping model. 113 strategy activities including traffic safety programmes for schools (Tziotis, 1994) audit of school playgrounds, professional training, bicycle helmet promotion	✓	✓	✓	Multi-agencies Community groups Schools Retailers Garages	Controlled trial without randomisation I = Shire of Bulla pop 28,347 C = Shire of Melton pop 28,812 (1986 figures)	Mortality and morbidity data Observed behaviour Attitudes Knowledge Area-wide environmental changes	Evidence of achievement of 4 objectives of programme 1. Increased community awareness 2. Development of injury prevention strategies (113 programmes developed) 3. Hazard reduction (>50% recommendation of schools playground safety audit enacted). 4. Increased use of safety helmets, devices and equipment, smoke detectors, safety seats. Little evidence of reduction of injury morbidity. Some evidence from telephone survey of reduction in minor injuries	Evidence of **Good*** quality *Partially effective* Good, well-documented study looking at process, impact and outcome measures. Longer follow-up needed

Table 21 (5) Community-based studies

Author, date & country	Injury target group & setting	Aims & content of intervention	Ed	Env	Leg	Healthy alliances	Study type & sample size	Outcome measures	Key results	Quality of evidence and effectiveness
(a) Ytterstad & Wasmuth (1995) Norway	(a) General population but specific components targeted at children	Harstad injury prevention study Comprehensive community-wide injury prevention programme, followed up over 7–9 years	✓	✓	✓	Wide range of organisations health and local authority, police, schools, private industry	(a) Controlled trial without randomisation I= 22,000 pop C=134,000 pop	(a) Mortality & morbidity data (hospital & primary care) police records	(a) 27% reduction in overall traffic injury rate. Significant reductions for children under 10 years and 15–24 years. *But* significant increase in injuries to elderly drivers. The reported 85% decrease in motor cycle injuries was associated with halving of local motor cycling exposure	Evidence of **Reasonable** quality *Partially effective/ inconclusive* in some age groups Non-equivalent control area with absent numerical data. ? Complete outcome data in I
(b) Ytterstad (1995)	(b) General population but specific components targeted at children	(a,b) Number of targets including child pedestrians and cyclists. Interventions include infant car seat loan scheme, counselling, speed enforcement, lobbying for cycle paths					(b) Before-and-after study without control I= 22,000 pop C=134,000 pop	(b) Morbidity data (A & E hospital admissions)	(b) For children under 16 years 37% reduction in cyclist injuries and 54% reduction in pedestrian injuries but both probably associated with decreased exposure	(b) *Partially effective/ inconclusive* in some age groups No evidence outcomes attributable to intervention Non- equivalent control area with absent numerical data ? Complete outcome

Table 21 (6) Community-based studies

Author, date & country	Injury target group & setting	Aims & content of intervention	Ed	Env	Leg	Healthy alliances	Study type & sample size	Outcome measures	Key results	Quality of evidence and effectiveness
(c) Ytterstad & Sogaard (1995)	Children under 5 Community-wide	(c) Community-based intervention to prevent burns Interventions include parent counselling at routine child health visits, home visits, professional awareness raising, recommended devices	✔	✔			(c) Controlled trial without randomisation I=22,000 pop C_1 =134,000 pop C_2= 14,000 pop	(c) Morbidity & mortality (A & E hospital admissions)	(c) 53% reduction in burn injury rates in I community, 10% increase in C1 and 14% decrease in C2 Admissions in I in later period may have been for less severe injuries as bed days per patients and surgical procedures decreased	(c) *Effective* Non-equivalent control area ? Complete outcome data in I

References

Note: *evaluated studies included in Tables 4–21

Agran, P, Dunkle, D and Winn, D (1987). Effects of legislation on motor vehicle injuries to children. *Am J Dis Child* **141**:959.

Allsop, R and Turner, E (1986). Road casualties and public transport fares in London. *Accid Anal Prev* **18**:147.

Alpert, J J and Heagarty, M C (1966). Evaluation of a program for distribution of ipecac syrup for the emergency home management of poison ingestions. *J Pediatr* **69**:142–6

Alwash, R and McCarthy, M (1987). How do child accidents happen? *Health Education Journal* **46**(4):169.

Alwash, R and McCarthy, M (1988). Accidents in the home among children under 5: ethnic differences or social disadvantage? *BMJ* **296**:1450.

*Ampofo-Boateng, K, Thomson, J, Grieve, R, Pitcairn, T, Lee, D and Demetre, J (1992). A developmental and training study of children's ability to find safe routes to cross the road. *British Journal of Developmental Psychology* **83**(2):189–202, May.

*Antaki, C, Morris, P and Flude, B (1986). The effectiveness of the 'Tufty Club' in road safety education. *Br J Educ Psychol* **56**:363.

Avery, J and Jackson, R (1993). *Children and their accidents*. London: Edward Arnold.

Avery, J, Vaudin, J, Fletcher, J and Watson, J (1990). Geographical and social variations in mortality due to childhood accidents in England and Wales 1975–84. *Public Health* **104**:171.

Avery, J G and Gibbs, B (1985). Long term disability following accidents in childhood in *Proceedings of symposium on Accidents in Childhood*. Occasional Paper 7. London: Child Accident Prevention Trust.

Baltimore, C L and Meyer, R J (1968). A study of storage, child behavioral traits, and mothers' knowledge of toxicology in 52 poisoned families and 52 comparison families. *Pediatrics* **42**:312–17.

*Banbury, J (1992). *BBC Education. 'Play it Safe' 1. Evaluation of the broadcasts and back-up material*. BBC.

Barker, M and Power, C (1993). Unpublished paper reported in Woodroffe, Glicknem, Barker and Power.

*Barone, V J, Green, B F and Lutzker, J R (1986). Home safety with families being treated for child abuse and neglect. *Behav Modif* **10**(1):93–114.

Barry, W, Little and T, Sibert, J (1982). Childhood drownings in private swimming pools: an avoidable cause of death. *BMJ* **285**:542.

*Bass, J, Mehta, K, Ostrovsky, M and Halperin, S (1985). Educating parents about injury prevention. *Pediatric Clinics of North America* **32**(1):233.

*Bass, J, Mehta, K and Ostrovsky, M (1991). Childhood injury prevention in a suburban Massachusetts population. *Public Health Reports* **106**(4):437.

Bass, J L, Cristoffel, K K, Widome, M, Boyle, W, Scheidt, P, Stanwick, R and Roberts, K (1993). Childhood injury prevention counseling in primary care settings: a critical review of the literature. *Pediatrics* **92**(4):544–80.

*Bass, L W and Wilson, T R (1964). The pediatrician's influence in private practice measured by a controlled seat belt study. *Pediatrics* **33**:700–4.

*Baudier, F, Marchais, M, Ferry, B, Bourderont, D, Pinochet, C and Blum, D (1988). Programme coopératif de prévention des accidents domestiques de l'enfant dans le département du Doubs. *Arch Fr Pediatr* **45**:499–503.

*Berger, L, Saunders, S, Armitage, K and Schauer, L (1984). Promoting the use of car safety devices for infants: an intensive health education approach. *Pediatrics* **74**(1):16.

*Bergman, A, Rivara, F, Richards, D and Rogers, L (1990). The Seattle children's bicycle helmet campaign. *Am J Dis Child* **144**:727.

Bjärås, G (1987). Experiences in local community activities in Sweden: the Sollentuna project. Proceedings of the Health Community: Child Safety as part of health promotion activities conference, Stockholm, April.

Bouter, L M, van Rijn, O J L and Kok, G (1990). Importance of planned health education for burn injury prevention. *Burns* **16**(3):198–202.

*Bowman, J, Sanson-Fisher, R and Webb, G (1987). Interventions in preschools to increase the use of safety restraints by preschool children. *Pediatrics* **79**(1):103.

*Boxall, J (1988). School crossing patrols: How effective are they? *Traffic Engineering + Control* (Nov):586.

Boyle, W E , Bull, M, Katcher, M L *et al.* (1994). Office based counseling for injury prevention. *Pediatrics* **94**(4):566.

*Bryan-Brown, K. (1994). *The effectiveness of the General Accident Eastern Region Children's Traffic Club*. Project Report 99. Crowthorne: Transport Research Laboratory.

*Bryan-Brown, K (1995). The effects of a children's traffic club. In: Department of Transport: *Road Accidents Great Britain, 1994*.

*Cameron, M, Heiman, L and Neiger, D (1992). *Evaluation of the Bicycle Helmet Wearing Law in Victoria during its first 12 months*. Victoria, Australia: Accident Research Centre, Monash University.

*Cameron, M H, Vulcan, A P, Finch, C F and Newstead, S V (1994). Mandatory bicycle helmet use following a decade of helmet promotion in Victoria, Australia – an evaluation. *Accid Anal Prev* **26**(3):325–37.

Carlsson, G, Norin, H and Ysander, L (1991). Rearward-facing child seats – the safest car restraint for children? *Accid Anal Prev.* **23** (2/3):175–82.

Cass, D, Ross, F and Gratton-Smith, T (1991). Child drowning: a changing pattern. *Med J Aust* (Feb 4) **154**:163–65.

Centre for Reviews and Dissemination (1995). *Review of the research on the effectiveness of Health Service interventions to reduce variations in health*. CRD Report 3. University of York.

Chafee-Bahamon, C and Lovejoy, F H, Jr (1983). Effectiveness of a Regional Poison Center in reducing excess emergency room visits for children's poisonings. *Pediatrics* **72**:164–9.

*Chang, A, Dillman, A S, Leonard, E and English, P (1985). Teaching car passenger safety to preschool children. *Pediatrics* **76**:425–8.

Child Accident Prevention Trust (1988). *The safety of children in cars*. Occasional Paper No. 9. London: CAPT.

Child Accident Prevention Trust (1989). *Basic principles of child accident prevention: a guide to action.* London: CAPT.

Child Accident Prevention Trust (1992). *The NHS and social costs of children's accidents: a pilot study.* London: CAPT.

Christian, M and Bullimore, D (1989). Reduction in accident severity in rear seat passengers using restraints. *Injury* **20**(5):262.

*Christophersen, E and Sullivan, M A (1982). Increasing the protection of newborn infants in cars. *Pediatrics* **70**:21–5.

*Christophersen, E R (1985). Enhancing the effectiveness of health education strategies. *Clinics in Perinatology* **12**:381–9.

Coleman, P, Harper, R, Kent, G, Munro, J, Nicholl, J P and Wild, D (1994). *The effectiveness of intervention strategies to prevent accidental injuries to adolescents and young adults aged 15–24 years in the UK.* Department of Health. Medical Care Research Unit, University of Sheffield.

*Colletti, R (1986). Longitudinal evaluation of a statewide network of hospital programs to improve child passenger safety. *Pediatrics* **77**(4):523.

*Colver, A, Hutchinson, P and Judson, E (1982). Promoting children's home safety. *BMJ* **285**:1177.

Colver, A and Pearson, P (1985). Safety in the home: How well are we doing? *Health Visitor* **58**:41.

Condie, C, Rivara, F P and Bergman, A B (1993). Strategies of a successful campaign to promote the use of equestrian helmets. *Public Health Rep* **108**(1):121–6.

Consumers Association' (1986). Report of the Consumers' Association's findings on the use of extendable (coiled) kettle flexes. *Which? Magazine* Dec:580–1.

*Coté, T, Sacks, J, Lambert-Huber, D *et al* (1992). Bicycle helmet use among Maryland children: effect of legislation and education. *Pediatrics* **89**(6):1216.

*Cushman, R, Down, J, MacMillan, N and Waclawik, H (1991). Helmet promotion in the emergency room following a bicycle injury: a randomized trial. *Pediatrics* **88**(1):43.

*Cushman, R, James, W and Waclawik, H (1991). Physicians promoting bicycle helmets for children: a randomized trial. *Am J Public Health* **81**(8):1044.

Dannenburg, A L, Gielen, A C, Beilenson, P L, Wilson, M H and Joffe, A (1993). Bicycle helmet laws and educational campaigns: an evaluation of strategies to increase children's helmet use. *Am J Public Health* **83**(5):667–74.

*Davidson, L L, Durkin, M S, Kuhn, L, O'Connor, P, Barlow, B and Heagarty, M C (1994). The impact of Safe Kids/Healthy Neighbourhoods injury prevention program in Harlem, 1988 through 1991. *Am J Public Health* **84**:580–6.

*Decker, M, Dewey, M, Hutcheson, R and Schaffner, W (1984). The use and efficacy of child restraint devices: the Tennessee experience, 1982 and 1983. *Journal of the American Medical Association* **252**(18):2571.

Deeks, J J, Glanville, J M, Sheldon, T A and Song, F (1995). *Undertaking systematic reviews of research on effectiveness: CRD guidelines for those carrying out or commissioning reviews.* CRD Report 4. University of York.

Dejeammes, M, Tingvall, C and Nygren, A (1986). *Effectiveness of child restraint laws.* Proceedings of an OECD workshop on the effectiveness of safety belt use law: a multinational examination.Washington, USA: Department of Transportation.

*Demetre, J, Lee, D, Grieve, R, Pitcairn, T, Ampofo-Boateng, K and Thomson, J (1992). Young children's learning on road-crossing simulations. *British Journal of Psychology* **83**(2):189–202.

Department of Health (1992). *The health of the nation: a strategy for health in England.* London: HMSO.

Department of Health (1993). *The health of the nation. Key area handbooks: Accidents.* London: Department of Health.

Department of the Environment (1991). *The building regulations. Glazing – materials and protection.* HMSO, Department of the Environment and Welsh Office.

Department of Trade and Industry (1986). *The prevention of accidents in and around the home: review of the role and effectiveness of publicity.* Consumer Safety Unit, DTI.

*Department of Trade and Industry (1989). *Hazard dome evaluation.* Cleverdon Steer Ltd for DTI, p. 281.

Department of Trade and Industry (1991). *Child safety equipment for use in the home.* London: DTI, Home and Leisure Accident Research.

Department of Trade and Industry (1992a). *Home and leisure accident research: 1989 data.* HASS Report. London: Consumer Unit, DTI.

*Department of Trade and Industry (1992b). *Giant safety trailer.* Research Report 282. SDG Research for DTI.

Department of Transport (1987). *Road safety: the next steps.* London: Department of Transport.

Department of Transport (1990). *Children and roads: a safer way.* London: Department of Transport.

Department of Transport (1992). *Killing speed and saving lives: the Government's strategy for tackling the problem of excess speed on our roads.* London: Department of Transport.

Department of Transport (1993). *Road traffic accidents Great Britain 1992. The casualty report.* London: HMSO.

*Dershewitz, R (1979). Will mothers use free household safety devices? *Am J Dis Child* **133**:61.

*Dershewitz, R and Williamson, J (1977). Prevention of childhood household injuries: a controlled clinical trial. *Am J Public Health* **67**(12):1148.

*Dershewitz, R A and Paichel, W (1984). Effectiveness of a health education programme in a lower socio economic population: replication of an Ipecac guidance study. *Clin Pediatr (Phila)* **23**(12):686–688.

*Dershewitz, R A, Posner, M K and Paichel, W (1983). The effectiveness of health education on home use of Ipecac. *Clin Pediatr (Phila)* **22**:268–70.

*DiGuiseppi, C, Rivara, F, Koepsell, T and Polissar, L (1989). Bicycle helmet use by children: evaluation of a community-wide helmet campaign. *Journal of the American Medical Association* **262**(16):2256.

*Doldissen, A and Draeger, W (1990). Environmental traffic management strategies in Buxterhude, West Germany. In: Tolley, R, ed. *The greening of urban transport.* London: Bellhaven, p. 266.

Dorsch, M M, Woodward, A J and Somers, R L (1987). Do bicycle safety helmets reduce the severity of head injuries in real crashes? *Accid Anal and Prev* **19**:183–90.

Downing, C (1987). *Evaluation of the impact and penetration of a children's traffic club.* Second International Conference on Road Safety, Groningen.

*Downing, C and Franklin, J (1989). *An evaluation of two local infant restraint loan schemes.* First World Conference on Accident and Injury Prevention; second conference on Child Accident Prevention, Stockholm.

*Downing, C S, Murray, G and Durrow, C (1981). *Effects of a road safety booklet for a pre-school traffic club.* Lab Report 992. Crowthorne: Department of Transport TRRL.

Dowswell, T, Jarvis, S and Towner, E (1994). *Reducing childhood accidents: the effectiveness of health promotion interventions. An annotated bibliography.* Newcastle: Northern and Yorkshire Regional Health Authority.

Dugdill, L and Ashton, J (1991). *Evaluation of the YUK Accidental Poisoning Prevention Campaign in Liverpool.* University of Liverpool, Department of Public Health.

*Eckelt, K, Fannon, M, Blades, B and Munster, A (1985). A successful burn prevention program in elementary schools. *J Burn Care Rehabil* **6**(6):509.

*Elberg, J J, Schroder, H A, Glent-Madsen L and Hall, K V (1987). Burns: epidemiology and the effect of a prevention programme. *Burns* **13**(5):391–3.

*Engel, U (1982). *'Short term' and area wide evaluation of safety measures implemented in a residential area named Osterbro: a case study.* Seminar on short-term and area-wide evaluation of safety measures. Amsterdam.

*Erdmann, T, Feldman, K, Rivara, F, Heimbach, M and Wall, H (1991). Tap water burn prevention: the effect of legislation. *Pediatrics* **88**(3):572.

Evans, L (1991). *Traffic safety and the driver.* New York: Van Nostrand Reinhold.

*Fallat, M E and Rengers, S J (1993). The effect of education and safety devices on scald burn prevention. *Journal of Trauma* **34**(1): 560–3; discussion 563–4.

Ferguson, J A, Sellar, C and Goldacre, M J (1992). Some epidemiological observations on medicinal and nonmedicinal poisoning in preschool children. *Journal Epidemiology and Community Health* **46**:207–10.

Fergusson, D and Horwood, L (1984). Risks of drowning in fenced and unfenced domestic swimming pools. *NZ Med J* **97**:777.

Fergusson, D M, Horwood, L J, Beautrais, A L and Shannon, F T (1982). A controlled field trial of poisoning prevention methods. *Pediatrics* **69**:(5)515–20.

*Finch, C F, Heiman, L and Neiger, D (1992). *Bicycle use and helmet wearing rates in Melbourne 1987–1992: the influence of the Helmet Wearing Law.* Victoria, Australia: Accident Research Centre, Monash University.

*Finch, C F, Newstead, S V, Cameron, M H and Vulcan, A P (1993). *Head injury reduction in Victoria 2 years after introduction of mandatory bicycle helmet use.* Report 51. Victoria, Australia: Monash University Accident Research Centre.

Finney, J W, Christophersen, E R, Frisman, P C, Kalnins, I V, Maddox, J E, Peterson, L et al. (1993). Society of Pediatric Psychology Task Force Report: pediatric psychology and injury control. *J Ped Psych* **18**(4):499–526.

Finocchiaro, C and Torpey, S (1989). Process evaluation of the bassinet restraint loan scheme in Victoria. *Australian Pediatric Journal* **25**:270–3.

Firth, D (1973). *The road safety aspects of the Tufty Club.* Department of Transport. Transport and Road Research Laboratory.

Fisher, L, Godard Harris, V, Van Buren, J, Quinn, J and DeMaio, A (1980). Assessment of a pilot child playground injury prevention project in New York State. *Am J Public Health* **70**(9):1000.

Foxcroft, D R, Lister-Sharp, D and Lowe, G (1996). *Review of effectiveness of health promotion interventions: young people and alcohol misuse.* London: Health Education Authority (in preparation).

Gallagher, S, Hunter, P and Guyer, B (1985). A home injury prevention program for children. *Pediatric Clinics of North America* **32**(1):95.

*Gallagher, S S, Messenger, K P and Guyer, B (1987). State and local responses to children's injuries: the Massachusetts Statewide Childhood Injury Prevention Program. *J Social Issues* **43**:149–62.

Gardiner, S, Smeeton, W, Koelmeyer, T and Cairns, F (1985). Accidental drownings in Auckland children. *NZ Med J* **98**(783):579.

Garraway, W, Macleod, D and Sharp, J (1991). Rugby injuries: the need for case registers. *BMJ* **303**:1082.

*Geddis, D and Pettengell, R (1982). Parent education: its effect on the way children are transported in cars. *NZ Med J* **95**(May):314.

*Geddis, D C and Appleton, I C (1986). Establishment and evaluation of a pilot car child seat rental scheme in New Zealand. *Pediatrics* **77**(2):167–72.

Gloag, D (1988). Strategies for accident prevention: a review of the present position. In: *Strategies for accident prevention: a colloquium.* Depatment of Health and Social Security, p. 65.

*Goodson, J, Buller, C and Goodson,W (1985). Prenatal child safety education. *Obstetrics and Gynaecology* **65**:312.

Gorman, R, Charney, E, Holtzman, N and Roberts, K (1985). A successful city-wide smoke detector giveaway program. *Pediatrics* **75**(1):14.

Graham, I and Svanström, L (1989). *Application to become a member of the safe community network.* White Report 276, Karolinska Institutet, Sundyberg. Glasgow: Castlemilk.

Graitcer, P L, Kellermann and Cristoffel, T (1995). A review of educational and legislative strategies to promote bicycle helmets. *Injury Prevention* 122–9.

*Grant, E, Turney, E, Bartlett, M, Winbon, C and Peterson, H D (1992). Evaluation of a burn prevention program in a public school system. *J Burn Care Rehabil* **13**:703–7.

Grayson, G (1981). The identification of training objectives: what shall we tell the children? *Accid Anal Prev* **13**(3):169.

Grayson, G and Howarth, C (1982). Evaluating pedestrian safety programmes. In: Chapman, A, Wade, F, Foo, H, eds. *Pedestrian Accidents.* Chichester: John Wiley, p. 109.

*Greenberg, L W and Coleman, A B (1982). A prenatal and postpartum safety education program: influence on parental use of infant car restraints. *J Dev Behav Pediatr* **3**:32–4.

*Gregersen, N P and Nolen, S (1994). Children's road safety and the strategy of voluntary traffic safety clubs. *Accid Anal Prev.* **26**(4): 463–70.

*Guerin, D and MacKinnon, D (1985). An assessment of the California child passenger restraint requirement. *Am J Public Health* **75**(2):142.

*Gundy, C M (1988). The effectiveness of a combination of police enforcement and public information for improving seat belt use. In: Rottengatter, J and de Bruin, R, eds. *Road user behaviour: theory and research.* Maastricht: van Gorum.

*Guyer, B, Gallagher, S, Chang, B, Azzara, C, Cupple, L and Colton, T (1989). Prevention of childhood injuries: evaluation of the Statewide Childhood Injury Prevention Program (SCIPP). *Am J Public Health* **79**(11):1521.

Hammarström, A (1989). Experience from a local safety project. Paper presented at the Conference on Child Accident Prevention, Stockholm 21–22 September 1989.

*Hammond, J and Varas, R (1990). Co-ordinated strategies in burn prevention programs; a case study. *J Burn Care Rehabil* **11**(4):376–78.

Harland, D (1992). Road safety education – the good practice project. In *Roads: the Journal of the Institute of Road Safety Officers* **14**(2).

*Harland, D G, Murray, G and Tucker, S (1991). Road safety education: making safe connections. Paper presented at Safety '91, Transport and Road Research Laboratory, Crowthorne.

Harland, G and Tucker, S (1994). 'Let's Decide – Walk Wise' – the development and testing of a pedestrian training resource. Paper presented at the 14th Conference of the British Health and Safety Society.

Hennessy, M, Arnold, R and Harvey, P (1994). *The first three years: final report of the first three years of the Shire of Bulla's Safe Living Program (1991–1993)*. Project Report. Shire of Bulla, Victoria.

Hillman, M (1993). *Cycle helmets: the case for and against*. London: Policy Studies Institute.

Hillman, M, Adams, J and Whitelegg, J (1990). *One false move: a study of children's independent mobility*. London: Policy Studies Institute.

*Hletko, P J, Robin, S S, Hletko, J D and Stone, M (1987). Infant safety seat use: reaching the hard to reach. *Am J Dis Child* **141**:1301–4.

Hollwarth, M E (1994). Speed limit of 30 Km/h as accident prevention for children. Tempo 30 aus der Sicht des Österreichischen Komitees für Unfallverhütung in Kindesalter. *Pédiatrie und Pédologie* **29**(2):A27–A29.

Home Office (1992). *Smoke alarms: incidence of ownership*. London: Home Office.

Home Office (1993). *Criminal statistics: England and Wales 1992*. London: HMSO.

Howarth, C and Gunn, M (1982). Pedestrian safety and the law. In: Chapman, A, Wade, F and Foot, H, eds. *Pedestrian accidents*. Chichester: John Wiley, p. 265.

Illingworth, C (1977). Playground equipment injuries. In: Jackson, R, ed. *Children, the environment and accidents*. London: Pitman Medical, p. 121.

Illingworth, C (1992). The argument for helmets. *BMJ* **305**:882.

Institute of Highways and Transportation (1993). Guidelines for urban safety management, IHT, 1990. *J Trauma* **34**:560–4.

Jackson, R H (1977). *Children, the environment and accidents*. London: Pitman Medical.

*Jämark, S, Ljungblom, B A and Turbell, T (1988). *Infant carriers – a trial in two counties*. VTI Report 316A. Linköping, Sweden: Swedish Road and Traffic Research Institute.

*Janssen, S (1991). Road safety in urban districts: final results of accident studies in the Dutch demonstration projects of the 1970s. *Traffic Engineering + Control*, p. 292.

Jarvis, S, Towner, E and Dowswell, T (1994). *Reducing childhood accidents . The effectiveness of health promotion interventions. A review of research methodologies*. Newcastle: Northern and Yorkshire Regional Health Authority.

*Jeffs, D, Booth, D and Calvert, D (1993). Local injury information, community participation and injury reduction. *Aust J Public Health* **17**:365–72.

Johnson, Z, Howell, F and Molloy, B (1993). Community mothers' programme: randomised controlled trial of non-professional intervention in parenting. *BMJ* **306**:1449–52.

Jones, D (1990). Child casualties in road accidents. In: *Road accidents: Great Britain 1989. The casualty report*. London: Department of Transport, p. 36.

Jones-Lee, M W (1993). Personnel willingness to pay for prevention: evaluating the consequences of accidents as a basis for preventive measures. *Addiction* **88**(7):913–21.

Jordan, E A, Duggan, A K and Hardy, J B (1993). Injuries in children of adolescent mothers: home safety education associated with decreased injury risk. *Pediatrics* **91**:481–7.

*Jørgensen, E (1985). Bicycle tracks in urban areas in Denmark. Evaluation of the effect on safety. In Biecheler, M, Lacombe, C and Muhlrad, N, eds. *Evaluation 85: Proceedings of the International Meeting on the evaluation of local traffic safety measures.* Paris, p. 755.

Katcher, M (1987). Prevention of tap water scald burns: evaluation of a multi-media injury control program. *Am J Public Health* **77**(9):1195.

*Katcher, M, Landry, G and Shapiro, M (1989). Liquid-crystal thermometer use in pediatric office counselling about tap water burn prevention. *Pediatrics* **83**(5):766–71.

*Kelly, B, Sein, C and McCarthy, P (1987). Safety education in a pediatric primary care setting. *Pediatrics* **79**(5):818.

Kemp, A and Sibert, J (1992). Drowning and near drowning in children in the United Kingdom: lessons for prevention. *BMJ* **304**:1143.

Kendrick, D (1994). Role of the primary health care team in preventing accidents to children. *British Journal of General Practice* **44**:372–5.

Kendrick, D and Marsh, P (1994). *The effectiveness of intervention programmes in reducing accidental injuries to children and young people: a literature review.* Report prepared for Trent Regional Health Authority.

Kimber, R (1990). Appropriate speeds for different road conditions. In: PACTS, ed. *Speed, accidents and injury: reducing the risks.* London: PACTS.

King, K and Ball, D (1989). *A holistic approach to accident and injury prevention in children's playgrounds.* London: LSS.

King, D, Lawson, S, Proctor, S and Hoyland, M (1987). *Child pedestrian accidents in inner areas: patterns and treatment.* PTRC Summer Annual Meeting. University of Bath.

Klang, M, Andersson, R and Lindquist, K (eds) (1993). *Safe communities: The application to industrialised countries.* Lindköping Collaborating Centre, Occasional Paper 5. Special Issue, Report from a seminar in Lindköping 26–27 November 1990, Department of Community Medicine, University of Lindköping. Reported in Popay and Young (1993).

Klassen, T P (1995). *The effectiveness of injury control interventions.* MSc thesis, McMaster University, Hamilton, Ontario, Canada.

*Kraus, J (1985). Effectiveness of measures to prevent unintentional deaths of infants and children from suffocation and strangulation. *Public Health Reports* **100**(2):231.

*Kravitz, H and Grove, M (1973). Prevention of accidental falls in infancy by counselling mothers. *Illinois Medical Journal* **144**(6):570.

*Krug, A, Ellis, J B, Hay, I T, Mokgabudi, N F and Robertson, J (1994). The impact of child resistant containers in the incidence of paraffin (kerosene) ingestion in children. *S Afr Med J* **84**(11):730–4.

*Kuhn, L, Davidson, L L and Durkin, M S (1994). Use of Poisson regression and time series analysis for detecting changes over time in rates of child injury following a prevention program. *Am J Epidemiol* **140**(10):943–55.

*Laing, R M and Bryant, V (1991). Prevention of burn injuries to children involving nightwear. *N Z Med J* **104**:363.

Lawson, S and Edwards, P. The involvement of ethnic minorities in road accidents: data from three studies of young pedestrian casualties. *Traffic Engineering + Control* (January), p. 12.

Learmouth, A (1979). Factors in child burn and scald accidents in Bradford 1969–73. *Journal of Epidemiology and Community Health* **33**:270.

*Leicester, P, Nassam, F and Wise, A (1991). *The introduction of compulsory bicycle helmet wearing in Victoria*. Vic Roads report GR 91–4.

*Lewis, B, Kaplan, S and Weinberg, K (1994). Do children retain what they are taught? *J Burn Care Rehabil* **15**(3):298–302.

*Linares, A Z and Linares, H A (1979). Burn prevention programmes for children: are they effective? *Burns* **6**:73–9.

*Lindqvist, K S (1993). Does the use of child safety seats increase as a result of loan schemes? *Accid Anal Prev* **25**(4):421–9.

Lowne, R, Roberts, A, Roy, P, Hill, K and Jones, H (1984). *The effect of the UK seat belt legislation on restraint usage by children*. Society of Automotive Engineers.

Lynam, D and Harland, D (1992). *Child pedestrian safety in the UK*. Paper presented to the Forum of European Road Safety Research Institutes (FERSI).

Lynam, D, Mackie, A and Davies, C (1988). *Urban safety project: 1. Design and implementation of schemes*. Department of Transport, Transport and Road Research Laboratory.

*Mackay, A M and Rothman, K J (1982). The incidence and severity of burn injuries following Project Burn Prevention. *Am J Public Health* **72**(3):248–52.

Mackay, M (1987). Seat belt legislation in Britain. *J Trauma* **27**(7):759.

Mackie, A, Ward, H and Walker, R (1988). *Urban safety project. 2. Interim results for area wide schemes*. Department of Transport, Transport and Road Research Laboratory.

Mackie, A, Ward, H and Walker, R (1990). *Urban safety project. 3. Overall evaluation of area wide schemes*. Department of Transport, Transport and Road Research Laboratory.

*Macknin, M, Gustafson, C, Gassman, J and Barich, D (1987). Office education by pediatricians to increase seat belt use. *Am J Dis Child* **141**:1305.

Maimaris, C, Summers, C L, Browning, C and Palmer, C R (1994). Injury patterns in cyclists attending an accident and emergency department: a comparison of helmet wearers and no-wearers. *BMJ* **308**:1537–40.

*Maisel, G, Langdoc, B A, Jenkins, M Q and Aycock, E K (1967). Analysis of two surveys evaluating a project to reduce accidental poisoning amongst children. *Public Health Rep* **82**:555–60.

*Malenfant, F and Van Houten, R (1989). Increasing the percentage of drivers yielding to pedestrians in three Canadian cities with a multifaceted safety program. *Health Education Research* **5**(2):275–9.

Manciaux, M and Romer, C J (eds) (1991). *Accidents in childhood and adolescence. The role of research*. Geneva: World Health Organisation.

Mann, C N, Weller, S and Rauchschwalbe, R (1992). Bucket-related drownings in the United States, 1984 through 1990. *Pediatrics* **89**:1068.

Margolis, L, Wagenaar, A and Liu, W (1988). The effects of a mandatory child restraint law on injuries requiring hospitalization. *Am J Dis Child* **142**:1099.

Mathias, D and Colling, P (1988:). *An investigation into the asphyxiation of children due to inhalation of pen tops (PENTOPS)*. Department of Trade and Industry.

Matthews, J R, Friman, P C, Barone, V J, Ross, L V and Christophersen, E R (1987). Decreasing dangerous infant behaviors through parent instruction. *J Appl Behav Anal* **20**: 165–9.

McCabe, M and Moore, H (1990). Is National Fire Safety Week a waste of time? *Fire Prevention* **232**(September):12.

McCarthy, M (1991). Pedal cyclists, crash helmets and risk. *Public Health Reports* **105**:327.

McCarthy, M (1992). Do cycle helmets prevent serious head injury? *BMJ* **305**:881.

*McDermott, F T (1995). Bicyclist head injury prevention by helmets and mandatory wearing legislation in Victoria, Australia. *Ann R Coll Surg Engl* **77**(1):38–44.

McIntire, M, Angle, C, Ekins, B, Mofenson, H, Rauber, A and Schertz, R (1983). Trends in childhood poisoning: a collaborative study 1970, 1975, 1980. *Journal of Toxicology and Clinical Toxicology* **84**(21 (3)): 321–31.

*McLoughlin, E, Healer, C and Crawford, J (1979). Burn education intervention: a controlled study. *Burns* **6**:26–9.

*McLoughlin, E, Marchone, M, Hanger, L, German, P and Baker, S (1985). Smoke detector legislation: its effect on owner-occupied homes. *Am J Public Health* **75**(8):858.

*McLoughlin, E, Vince, C J, Lee, A M and Crawford, J D (1982). Project Burn Prevention: outcome and implications *Am J Public Health* **72**(3)241–7.

Mickalide, A (1991). Evaluation of the SAFE KIDS bicycle helmet campaign: Grassroots efforts increase helmet sales and use. *Childhood Injury Prevention Quarterly* (Winter):10.

*Miller, J R and Pless, I B (1977). Child automobile restraints: evaluation of health education. *Pediatrics* **59**:907–11.

*Miller, R, Reisinger, K, Blatter, M and Wucher, F (1982). Pediatric counselling and subsequent use of smoke detectors. *Am J Public Health* **74**(4):392.

Milliner, N, Pearn, J and Guard, R (1980). Will fenced pools save lives? A 10-year study from Mulgrave Shire, Queensland. *Med J Aust* **2**:510.

Mills, P J (1989). *Pedal cycle accidents – a hospital based study.* Transport and Road Research Laboratory Research Report 220. Crowthorne: TRRL.

Minchom, P, Sibert, J, Newcombe, R and Bowley, M (1984). Does health education prevent childhood accidents? *Postgraduate Medical Journal* **60**(April):260.

Moller, J (1995). An introduction to community based injury prevention. In: Ozanne-Smith, J and Williams, F. *Injury research and prevention: a text.* Clayton, Victoria: Monash University Accident Research Centre.

Morgan, M and Shute, R (1990). Smoking education and peer group influence. In: Foot, H, Morgan, M and Shute, R, eds. *Children helping children.* Chichester: John Wiley, pp. 307–26.

*Morris, B and Trimble, N (1991). Promotion of bicycle helmet use among schoolchildren: a randomized clinical trial. *Canadian Journal of Public Health* **82**(March/April):92.

Morris, B A P, Trimble, N E and Fendley, S J (1994). Increasing bicycle helmet use in the community. *Can Fam Physician* **40**:1126–31.

*Morrow, R (1989). A school-based program to increase seatbelt use. *J Family Practice* **29**:517–20.

*Morton, J G and Burton, J F (1979). An evaluation of the effectiveness of mouthguards in high-school rugby players. *N Z Dent J* **75**:151–3.

Mulligan, J, Law, C and Speller, V (1995). *Interventions to control injury in children and young people: a literature review.* Wessex Institute of Public Health Medicine. Final draft.

Munro, J, Coleman, P, Nicholi, J, Harper, R, Kent, G and Wild, D (1995). Can we prevent accidental inury to adolescents? A systematic review of the evidence. *Injury Prevention* **1**:249–55.

Mynors, P and Savell, A (1992). *Cycling on the Continent.* London: Local Authority Cycle Planning Group, Travers Morgan Transport.

Naidoo, J (1984). *Evaluation of the Play it Safe! campaign in Bristol*. Child Accident Prevention Trust.

National Committee for Injury Prevention and Control (1989). *Injury prevention: meeting the challenge*. New York: Oxford University Press.

National Fire Protection Association (1990). *US experience with smoke detectors: Who has them? How well do they work? When don't they work?* National Fire Protection Association.

National Safety Council of Australia (1992). *Community based injury prevention: a practical guide*. South Australia: National Safety Council of Australia.

*Neuwelt, E, Coe, M, Wilkinson, A and Avolio, A (1989). Oregon head and spinal cord injury prevention program and evaluation. *Neurosurgery* **24**(3):453.

*Nielsen, O (1990). Safe routes to school in Odense, Denmark. In: Tolley, R, ed. *The greening of urban transport*. London: Bellhaven, p. 255.

*Nishioka, N, Ieda, S, Takahashi, H *et al.* (1991). An experimental study on the safety behavior of children in a dashing-out situation – effects of verbal instructions and traffic conditions on safety behavior. *IATSS Research* **15**(1):39.

Nutbeam, D, Smith, C and Catford, J (1990). Evaluation in health education. A review of progress, possibilities and problems. *J Epidemiol and Community Health* **44**:83–9.

O'Reilly, D (1994). Child pedestrian safety in Great Britain. In: Road Safety Division, Department of Transport *Road accidents Great Britain 1993: the casualty report*. London: HMSO.

Oakley, A and Fullerton, D (1995). *Review of effectiveness of health promotion interventions to prevent accidents in the elderly*. Report prepared for the Health Education Authority, February 1995. Unpublished.

Oakley, A, Fullerton, D, Holland, J, Arnold, S, France-Dawson, M, Kelley, P and McGrellis, S (1995). Sexual health education interventions for young people: a methodological review. *BMJ* **310**:158–62.

Office of Population Censuses and Surveys (1988). *Occupational mortality: childhood supplement*. OPCS, Series DS. London: HMSO.

Office of Population Censuses and Surveys (1989). *General household survey 1987*. HMSO.

Office of Population Censuses and Surveys (1990). *General household survey 1988*. HMSO.

Office of Population Censuses and Surveys (1991). *General household survey 1989*. HMSO.

Office of Population Censuses and Surveys (1994). *1992 Mortality statistics: childhood. England and Wales*. London: HMSO.

*Olds, D L, Henderson, C R and Kitzman, H (1994). Does prenatal and infancy nurse home visitation have enduring effects on qualities of parental caregiving and child health at 25 to 50 months of life? *Pediatrics* **93**:89–98.

Organisation for Economic Co-operation and Development (1978). *Chairman's report and report of sub-group III: Mass media communication for pedestrian safety*. Crowthorne: Department of the Environment Transport and Road Research Laboratory.

*Ozanne-Smith, J, Sherrard, J, Brumen, I A and Vulcan, P (1994). *Community based injury prevention evaluation report. Shire of Bulla Safe Living Program*. Report 66. Victoria, Australia: Monash University Accident Research Centre.

Palmisano, P A (1981). Targeted intervention in the control of accidental drug overdoses by children. *Public Health Reports* **96**(2) 151–6.

*Parkin, P C, Spence, L J, Hu, X, Kranz, K E, Shortt, L G and Wesson, D E (1993). Evaluation of a promotional strategy to increase bicycle helmet use by children. *Pediatrics* **91**(4):772–7.

Parliamentary Advisory Council for Transport Safety (1992). *Road accidents in focus.* Briefing papers. London: PACTS.

Patrick, M, Bint, M and Pearn, J (1979). Saltwater drowning and near drowning accidents involving children. *Med J Aust* **i**:61–4.

*Paul, C L, Sanson-Fisher, R W, Redman, S and Carter, S (1994). Preventing accidental injury to young children in the home using volunteers. *Health Promotion International* **9**(4):241–9.

Pearn, J and Nixon, J (1977). Prevention of childhood drowning accidents. *Med J Aust* **1**:616.

*Prendergast, R, Ashworth, C, DuRant, R and Litaker, M (1992). Correlates of children's bicycle helmet use and short-term failure of school-level interventions. *Pediatrics* **19**(3):354.

*Penna, C and Lambert (1994). *'Streets Ahead' Evaluation.* Vic Roads. Report GR 94–13, Victoria.

Peterson, L (1988). Preventing the leading killer of children: the role of the school psychologist in injury prevention. *School Psychology Review* **17**:593–600.

Pharoah, T and Russell, J (1989). *Traffic calming: policy and evaluations in three European countries* Occasional Paper. London: South Bank Polytechnic.

Pitt, W (1986). Increasing incidence of childhood immersion injury in Brisbane. *Med J Aust* **144**(June 23):683.

Pless, I (1991). *The science and art of injury prevention in childhood: perspectives from Britain and abroad.* London: Child Accident Prevention Trust.

Pless, I B (1993). *The scientific basis of childhood injury prevention. A review of the medical literature.* London: Child Accident Prevention Trust.

Popay, J and Young, A (1993). *Reducing accidental death and injury in children. A report produced for NWRHA.* Penultimate draft.

Preston, B (1972). Statistical analysis of child pedestrian accidents in Manchester and Salford. *Accid Anal Prev* **4**:323.

Preston, B (1990). Home zones – child's play for inner cities. *Town and Country Planning* (April):116.

Preston, B (1992). *Cutting pedestrian casualties: cost-effective ways to make walking safer.* London: Transport 2000.

*Preusser, D and Blomberg, R (1984). Reducing child pedestrian accidents through public education. *J Safety Research* **15**:47.

*Preusser, D and Lund, A (1988). And keep on looking: a film to reduce pedestrian crashes among 9 to 12 year olds. *J Safety Research* **19**:177.

Puczynski, M and Marshall, D A (1992). Helmets! All the pros wear them. *Am J Public Health* **146**:1465–7.

Quan, L, Gore, E, Wentz, K, Allen, J and Novack, A (1989). Ten-year study of pediatric drownings and near-drownings in King County, Washington: lessons in injury prevention. *Pediatrics* **83**(6):1035.

Race, K (1988). Evaluating pedestrian safety education materials for children ages five to nine. *Journal of School Health* **58**(7):277.

Reisinger, K and Williams, A (1978). Evaluation of programs designed to increase the protection of infants in cars. *Pediatrics* **62**(3):280.

*Reisinger, K, Williams, A, Wells, J, John, C, Roberts, T and Podgainy, H (1981). Effect of pediatricians' counselling on infant restraint use. *Pediatrics* **67**(2):201.

Rivara, F (1985). Traumatic deaths of children in the United States: currently available prevention strategies. *Pediatrics* **75**:456.

*Rivara, F, Booth, C, Bergman, A, Rogers, L and Weiss, J (1991). Prevention of pedestrian injuries to children: effectiveness of a school training program. *Pediatrics* **88**(4):770.

Roberts, H, Smith, S J and Bryce, C (1993). Prevention is better . . . *Sociology of Health and Illness* **15**,4.

*Roberts, M and Fanurik, D (1986). Rewarding elementary school children for their use of safety belts. *Health Psychol* **5**(3):185–96.

*Roberts, M, Fanurik, D and Wilson, D (1988). A community program to reward children's use of seat belts. *Am J Community Psychol* **16**(3):395.

*Robertson, L S (1986). Community injury control programs of the Indian Health Service: an early assessment. *Public Health Rep* **101**:632–7.

*Robertson, L S, Kelley, A B, O'Neill, B, Wixom, C W, Eiswirth, R S, Haddon, W, Jr (1974). A controlled study of the effect of television messages on safety belt use. *Am J Public Health* **64**(11):1071–80.

*Robitaille, Y, Legault, J, Abbey, H and Pless, B (1990). Evaluation of an infant car seat program in a low-income community. *Am J Dis Child* **44**:74.

Rottengatter, J (1981). The influence of instructional variables on the effectiveness of traffic education. *Accid Anal Prev* **13**(3):241.

Rourke, L L (1994). Bicycle helmet use among schoolchildren. *Can Fam Physician* **40**: 1116–24.

Royles, M (1994). *International literature review of cycle helmets.* Project Report 76. Crowthorne: Transport Research Laboratory.

Russell, J, Kresnow, M J and Brackbill, R (1994). The effect of adult belt laws and other factors on restraint use for children under age 11. *Accid Anal Prev* **26**(3): 287–95.

Sabey, B (1987). *Road accidents in childhood: the problem.* PACTS/CAPT Conference on Road Accidents in Childhood. London: PACTS/CAPT.

Sacks, J, Brantley, M, Holmgreen, M and Rochat, R (1992). Evaluation of an intervention to reduce playground hazards in Atlanta child-care centers. *Am J Public Health* **82**(3):429.

*Sahlin, Y and Lereim, I (1990). Accidents among children below school age. *Acta Paediatrica Scandinavia* **79**:691.

Sandels, S (1975). *Children in traffic.* (Revised ed.) Surrey: Elek Books.

Sargent, K and Sheppard, D (1974). *The development of the Green Cross Code.* Laboratory Report 6QS. Crowthorne: Department of the Environment, Transport and Road Research Laboratory.

*Schelp, L (1987). Community intervention and changes in accident pattern in a rural Swedish municipality. *Health Promotion* **2**(2):109.

*Schelp, L (1988). The role of organizations in community participation – prevention of accidental injuries in a rural Swedish municipality. *Social Science and Medicine* **26**(11):1087.

*Scherz, R G (1976). Restraint systems for the prevention of injury to children in automobile accidents. *Am J Public Health* **66**:451–6.

*Schioldborg, P (1976). *Children, traffic and traffic training: analysis of the children's traffic club.* Fifth Congress of the International Federation of Pedestrians. Geilo, Norway.

*Schlesinger, E, Dickson, D, Westaby, J, Lowen, L, Logrillo, V and Maiwald, A (1966). A controlled study of health education in accident prevention. The Rockland County child injury project. *Am J Dis Child* **3**(May):490.

*Schneider, M L, Ituarte, P and Stokols, D (1993). Evaluation of a community bicycle helmet promotion campaign: What works and why. *Am J Health Promotion* **7**(4):281–7.

*Schnell, L R and Tanz, R R (1993). The effect of providing ipecac to families seeking poison related services. *Pediatr Emerg Care* **9**(1):36–9.

*Schwarz, D F, Grisso, J A, Miles, C, Holmes, J H and Sutton, R L (1993). An injury prevention program in an urban African-American community. *Am J Public Health* **83**:675–80.

Seekins, T, Fawcett, S, Cohen, S *et al.* (1988). Experimental evaluation of public policy: the case of state legislation for child passenger safety. *J Appl Behav Anal* **21**(3):233.

*Sewell, C M, Hull, H F, Fenner, J, Graf, H and Pike, J (1986). Child restraint law effects on motor vehicle accident fatalities and injuries: the New Mexico experience. *Pediatrics* **78**(6)1079–84.

Shaw, K, McCormick, M, Kustra, S, Ruddy, R and Casey, R (1988). Correlates of reported smoke detector usage in an inner-city population: Participants in a smoke detector give-away program. *Am J Public Health* **78**(6):650.

Sheller, J P, Muchardt, O, Jonsson, B and Mikkelsen, M B (1995). Burn injuries caused by fireworks: effect of prophylaxis. *Burns* **21**(1):50–3.

*Sibert, J R, Clarke, A J and Mitchell, M P (1985). Improvements in child resistant containers. *Arch Dis Child* **60**:1155–7.

Sibert, J R, Craft, A W and Jackson, R H (1977). Child resistant packaging and accidental child poisoning. *Lancet* (6 August) 289–90.

Simon, J, Leven-Sohn, A, Metzger, B B, Hardman, S and Klein, S J (1993). Burn prevention through Weatherization Assistance Programs. *Am J Public Health* **82**(12):1787–8.

Singh, A and Spear, M (1989). *Road safety education in schools and colleges. Summary report.* Contractor Report 133. Transport and Road Research Laboratory.

Sinnott, W (1977). Safety aspects of domestic architecture. In: Jackson, R, ed. *Children, the environment and accidents.* London: Pitman Medical, p. 76.

*Sørensen, B (1976). Prevention of burns and scalds in a developed country. *J Trauma* **16**(4):249.

*Sowers-Hoag, K M, Thyer, B A and Bailey, J S (1987). Promoting automobile safety belt use in young children *J Appl Behav Anal* **20**:133–8.

Spaite, D, Murphy, M, Criss E, Valenzuela, T and Meislin, H (1991). A prospective analysis of injury severity among helmeted and non-helmeted bicyclists involved in collisions with motor vehicles. *J Trauma* **31**(4):1510.

*Spiegel, C and Lindaman, F (1977). Children can't fly: a program to prevent childhood morbidity and mortality from window falls. *Am J Public Health* **67**(12):1143.

Spyker, D (1985). Submersion injury: epidemiology, prevention and management. *Pediatric Clinics of North America* **32**(1):113.

Stevenson, T and Lennie, J (1992). Empowering school students in developmental strategies to increase bicycle helmet wearing. *Health Education Research* **7**(4):555–66.

Stone, D H (1993). *Accident prevention research – an overview. A selective review of the health literature, with special reference to Scotland.* Commissioned by Scottish Office Home and Health Department. Unpublished.

*Streff, F M, Molnar, L J and Christoff, C (1992). Increasing safety belt use in a secondary enforcement state: evaluation of a three-county special enforcement program. *Accid Anal Prev* **24**(4) 369–83.

*Stuy, M, Green, M and Doll, N (1993). Child care centers: a community resource for injury prevention. *J Dev Behav Pediatr* **14**(4):224–9.

*Sullivan, M, Cole, B, Lie, L and Twomey, J (1990). Reducing child hazards in the home: A joint venture in injury control. *J Burn Care Rehabil* **11**:(2)175–9.

*Tellnes, G (1985). An evaluation of an injury prevention campaign in general practice in Norway. *Family Practice* **2**(2):91.

Tengs, T O, Adams, M E, Pliskin, J S, Safran, D G, Siegel, J E, Weinstein, M C and Graham, J D (1995). 500 lifesaving interventions and their cost effectiveness. *Risk Analysis* **15**(3):369–90.

*Thomas, K, Hassanein, R and Christophersen, E (1984). Evaluation of group well-child care for improving burn prevention practices in the home. *Pediatrics* **74**(5):879.

Thomas, S, Acton, C, Nixon, J, Battistutta, D, Pit, W R and Clark, R (1994). Effectiveness of bicycle helmets in preventing head injury in children: case control study. *BMJ* **308**:173–6.

Thompson, J, Fraser, E and Howarth, C (1985). Driver behaviour in the presence of child and adult pedestrians. *Ergonomics* **28**(10):1469.

Thompson, R, Rivara, F and Thompson, D (1989). A case-control study of the effectiveness of bicycle safety helmets. *New England Journal of Medicine* **320**(21):1361.

*Thompson, R, Summers, S, Rampey-Dobbs R, Mani, M M, Hiebert, J H and Schneider, S (1992). The effect of instruction on burn prevention in eighth grade students in preparation for babysitting. *J. Burn Care Rehabil* **13**:482–6.

*Thomson, J, Ampofo-Boateng, K, Pitcairn, T, Grieve, R, Lee, D and Demetre, J (1992). Behavioural group training of children to find safe routes to cross the road. *Br J Educ Psychol* **62**:173.

Thomson, J A (1991). *The facts about child pedestrian accidents.* London: Cassell Educational.

Thuen, F and Mæland, J G (1993). Accident prevention activities in the Norwegian municipalities: the local response to a national campaign. *Scand J Soc Med* **21**(2):129–34.

*Thyer, B and Geller, E (1987). The 'Buckle-up' dashboard sticker. An effective environmental intervention for safety belt promotion. *Environment and Behaviour* **19**(4):484.

Tillman, M (1992). A study of the longer term effects of the urban safety project. The case of Reading, Berkshire (MSc Transport Operations Research Group). University of Newcastle upon Tyne.

Towner, E, Dowswell, T and Jarvis, S (1993). *Reducing childhood accidents. The effectiveness of health promotion interventions: a literature review.* London: Health Education Authority.

Towner, E, Jarvis, S N, Walsh, S S M and Aynsley-Green, A (1994). Measuring exposure to injury risk in schoolchildren aged 11–14. *BMJ* **308**(12):449–52.

Towner, E M L (1994). *Unintentional injuries in childhood. A review of the effectiveness of health education and health promotion.* Dutch Centre for Health Promotion and Health Education and IUPHE/EURO.

Towner, E M L (1995). The role of health education in childhood injury prevention. *Injury Prevention* **1**:53–8.

Towner, E M L and Jarvis, S N (1996). Unintentional injury prevention. In: David, T J (ed). *Recent Advances in Pediatrics* – 14. London: Churchill Livingstone.

Transport and Health Study Group. *Health on the move. Policies for health promoting transport*. London: Public Health Alliance, Transport and Road Research Laboratory,

Transport and Road Research Laboratory (1980). Cycle training: a TRRL investigation. *Traffic Education*, vol. 4. London: Transport and Road Research Laboratory.

Transport and Road Research Laboratory (1991). *Children should be seen and not hurt. Children and road traffic accidents*. Texaco Ltd.

Transport Research Laboratory (1992). *Restraint use by car occupants 1990–92*. TRL leaflet, LF2056. Crowthorne.

Trippe, H (1992). Helmets for pedal cyclists. *BMJ* **305**:843.

★Tucker, S (1992). The operation of the Eastern Region traffic club. In: *Working Paper WP/RUS/116*. Transport and Road Research Laboratory.

Tunbridge, R (1987). *An in-depth study of road accident casualites and their injury patterns*. Research Laboratory Report No. RR136. Crowthorne: Transport and Road Research Laboratory.

★Tziotis, M (1994). *Evaluation of the 'Safe Routes to Schools' and 'Walk with Care' Programs*. Vic Roads, Victoria.

van der Molen, H, van den Herik, and van der Klaauw, C (1983). Pedestrian behaviour of children and accompanying parents during school journeys: an evaluation of a training programme. *Br J Educ Psychol* **53**:152.

van Kernebeek, E (1992). *Sports injuries, how to prevent them. A nationwide health education campaign in the Netherlands 1988–92*. The Netherlands: Dutch Institute of Sports and Health and Consumer Safety Unit.

van Mechelen, W *et al.* (1993) Prevention of running injuries by warm-up, cool down, and stretching exercises. *Am J Sports Medicine* **21**(5):711–19.

★van Schagen, I N L G and Brookhuis, K A (1994). Training young cyclists to cope with dynamic traffic situations. *Accid Anal Prev* **26**(2):223–30.

★van Schagen, I (1988). Training children to make safe crossing decisions. In: Rottengatter, J and de Bruin, R, eds. *Road user behaviour: theory and research*. Maastricht: van Gorum.

★Varas, R, Carbone, R and Hammond, J S H (1988). A one-hour burn prevention program for grade school children: its approach and success. *J Burn Care Rehabil* **9**(1):69.

Vernberg, K, Culver-Dickinson, P and Spyker, D A (1984). The deterrent effect of poison warning stickers. *Am J Dis Child* **138**:1018–20.

Vimpani, G (1989). Injury surveillance: a key to effective control of childhood injuries. *Australian Paediatric Journal* **25**:10–13.

★Vulcan, A, Cameron, M and Watson, W (1992). Mandatory bicycle helmet use: experience in Victoria, Australia. *World Journal of Surgery* **16**:389.

★Wagenaar, A and Webster, D (1986). Preventing injuries to children through compulsory automobile safety seat use. *Pediatrics* **78**(4):662.

Walker, F, Booth, D, Southby, M and Long, K (1991). Using subjective data to evaluate ECIPP in Illawarra. *Health Promotion Journal of Australia* **1**(2):43–6.

★Walker, R and Gardner, J (1989). *Urban safety project: the Nelson scheme*. Department of Transport, Transport and Road Research Laboratory.

*Walker, R and McFetridge, M (1989). *Urban safety project: the Bradford scheme.* Department of Transport, Transport and Road Research Laboratory.

*Waller, A E, Clarke, J and Langley, J D (1993). An evaluation of a program to reduce home hot tap water temperatures. *Aust J Public Health* **17**:116.

Walton, W (1982). An evaluation of the poison prevention packaging act. *Pediatrics* **69**(3):363.

Ward, H, Cave, J, Morrison, A, Allsop, R and Evans, A (1994). *Pedestrian activity and accident risk.* Basingstoke: AA Foundation for Road Safety Research.

*Ward, H, Norrie, J, Sang, A and Allsop, R (1989a). *Urban safety project: the Reading scheme.* Department of Transport, Transport and Road Research Laboratory.

*Ward, H, Norrie, J, Sang, A and Allsop, R (1989b). *Urban safety project: the Sheffield scheme.* Department of Transport, Transport and Road Research Laboratory.

*Ward, H, Norrie, J, Allsop, R and Sang, A (1989c). *Urban safety project: the Bristol scheme.* Department of Transport, Transport and Road Research Laboratory.

Ward, H (1991). *Preventing road accidents to children: the role of the NHS.* London: Health Education Authority.

*Webne, S, Kaplan, B and Shaw, M (1989). Pediatric burn prevention: an evaluation of the efficacy of a strategy to reduce tap water temperature in a population at risk for scalds. *Dev Behav Pediatr* **10**(4):187.

Weiss, B (1992). Trends in bicycle helmet use by children: 1985 to 1990. *Pediatrics* **89**(1):78.

*West, R, Sammons, P and West, A (1993). Effects of a traffic club on road safety knowledge and self reported behaviour of young children and their parents. *Accid Anal Prev* **25**(5):609–18.

Whitehead, L and Curtis, L (1983). *How to watersafe infants and toddlers.* Tucson: HP Books.

Whitehead, M (1991). *Avoiding the pitfalls. Notes on the planning and implementation of health education strategies and the special role of the HEA.* London: Health Education Authority.

Whitelegg, J (1987). A geography of road traffic accidents. *Trans Institute of British Geographers* **12**:161.

Whitelegg, J and Davis, R (1992). Cycle helmets. *BMJ* **305**:504.

*Williams, A and Lund, A (1987). Results of a seat belt use law enforcement and publicity campaign in Elmira, New York. *Accid Anal Prev* **19**(4):243.

*Williams, H and Sibert, J (1983). *BMJ* **286**:1893.

Wilson, M, Baker, S, Tenet, S, Shock, S and Gabarius, S (1991). *Saving children. A guide to injury prevention.* Oxford: Oxford University Press.

Wintemute, G and Wright, M (1990). Swimming pool owners' opinions of strategies for prevention of drowning. *Pediatrics* **85**(1):63.

Wintemute, G, Drake, C and Wright, M (1991). Immersion events in residential swimming pools: evidence for an experience effect. *Am J Dis Child* **145**(Oct):1200.

Wols, M and Strange, G R (1993). Pediatric injury prevention annotated bibliography. *Ann Emerg Med* **22**(3):547.

*Wood, T and Milne, P (1988). Head injuries to pedal cyclists and the promotion of helmet use in Victoria, Australia. *Accid Anal Prev* **20**(3):177.

Woodroffe, C, Glickman, M, Barker, M and Power, C (1993). *Children, teenagers and health. The key data.* Bucks: Open University Press.

*Woolf, A, Lewander, W, Filippone, G and Lovejoy, F (1987). Prevention of childhood poisoning: efficacy of an educational program carried out in an emergency clinic. *Pediatrics* **80**:359–63.

*Woolf, A D, Saperstein, A and Forjuoh, S (1992). Poisoning prevention knowledge and practices of parents after a childhood poisoning incident. *Pediatrics* **90**(6):867–70.

*Wright, M, Rivara, F D and Ferse, D (1995). Evaluation of the Think First head and spinal cord injury prevention program. *Injury Prevention* **1**:81–5.

Yamamoto, L, Yee, A, Matthews, W and Wiebe, R (1992). A one-year series of pediatric ED water-related injuries: the Hawaii EMS-C project. *Pediatric Emergency Care* **8**(3):129.

*Yeaton, W and Bailey, J (1978). Teaching pedestrian safety skills to young children: an analysis and one-year follow up. *J Appl Behav Anal* **11**:315.

*Young, D and Lee, D (1987). Training children in road crossing skills using a roadside simulation. *Accid Anal Prev* **19**(5):327.

*Ytterstad, B (1995). The Harstad Injury Prevention Study: hospital-based injury recording used for outcome evaluation of community-based prevention of bicyclist and pedestrian injury. *Scand J Prim Health Care* **13**(2):141–9.

*Ytterstad, B and Sogaard, A J (1995). The Harstad Injury Prevention Study: prevention of burns in small children by a community based intervention. *Burns* **21**(4):259–66.

*Ytterstad, B and Wasmuth, H H (1995). The Harstad Injury Prevention Study: Evaluation of hospital-based injury recording and community-based intervention for traffic injury prevention. *Accid Anal Prev* **27**(1):111–23.